WEIGHT LOSS RECIPES COOKBOOK 2024

A Comprehensive Collection of Wholesome Recipes Tailored for Effortless Weight Loss and Sustainable Well-being

Milton B. Graham

CONTENTS

INTRODUCTION

Welcome to your transformation in 2024! This isn't just another weight loss cookbook; it's your culinary passport to a healthier, happier you. We understand the challenges of navigating food choices while aiming for weight loss. Forget bland restrictions and deprivation. This book unlocks a world of vibrant flavors and satisfying dishes that support your goals, without sacrificing taste or enjoyment.

Why 2024 is Your Year:

This year, weight loss isn't about fads or quick fixes. It's about sustainable, positive changes that fit seamlessly into your lifestyle. We've curated recipes that are:

- Modern and adaptable: Packed with trendy ingredients and global influences, these recipes cater to diverse palates and dietary preferences. From plant-based wonders to lean protein options, there's something for everyone.
- Quick and easy: Busy schedules don't have to derail your progress. We offer a variety of dishes perfect for weeknight meals, meal prepping, and on-the-go lunches.
- Nutrient-rich and balanced: Forget restrictive diets! These recipes are designed to nourish your body with essential vitamins, minerals, and fiber, keeping you energized and satisfied.
- Flavorful and exciting: Weight loss shouldn't mean sacrificing taste. We've crafted dishes that are bursting with flavor, using creative techniques and delicious combinations to keep your taste buds happy.

More than Just Recipes:

This book is your complete weight loss companion. We offer:

- Expert guidance: Registered dietitians and chefs provide insights on healthy eating, portion control, and mindful choices.
- Meal plans and tips: Get weekly meal suggestions tailored to different calorie needs and dietary preferences. Plus, discover helpful hacks and substitutions to personalize your journey.

Join the Movement: Losing weight shouldn't be a solitary journey. Share your culinary creations with our online community, swap tips, and celebrate each other's successes. We're here to support you every step of the way.

This cookbook is your key to unlocking a healthier, happier you in 2024. Let's embark on this delicious journey together, one flavorful bite at a time!

UNDERSTANDING WEIGHT LOSS AND NUTRITION

In our quest for healthier lifestyles, weight loss and nutrition stand as cornerstone elements. However, grasping the intricacies of these concepts is essential for achieving sustainable results. Let's delve into a deeper understanding of weight loss and nutrition, exploring their interplay and significance in our well-being.

Weight Loss: Weight loss refers to the reduction of body mass, typically involving a decrease in fat tissue. While many associate weight loss solely with aesthetic goals, its importance extends far beyond appearance. Maintaining a healthy weight is vital for overall health, as excess body fat can increase the risk of numerous chronic diseases, including diabetes, heart disease, and certain cancers.

Key Factors Influencing Weight Loss:

❖ Caloric Balance: Weight loss occurs when the calories consumed through food and beverages are fewer than those expended through metabolism and physical activity. This creates a calorie deficit, prompting the body to utilize stored fat for energy.

❖ Nutrition: The quality of calories consumed significantly impacts weight loss. Nutrient-dense foods, such as fruits, vegetables, lean proteins, and whole grains, provide essential vitamins, minerals, and fiber while promoting satiety. On the other hand, foods high in added sugars, unhealthy fats, and refined carbohydrates can contribute to weight gain and poor health outcomes.

❖ Physical Activity: Regular exercise plays a crucial role in weight loss by increasing calorie expenditure, improving metabolism, and enhancing overall health. Combining cardio exercises, strength training, and flexibility exercises can optimize weight loss and promote lean muscle mass.

❖ Behavior and Lifestyle: Behavior modifications, such as mindful eating, portion control, stress management, and adequate sleep, are integral to successful weight loss. Adopting sustainable lifestyle changes can help individuals overcome barriers and maintain long-term adherence to healthy habits.

Nutrition: Nutrition encompasses the intake of nutrients from food and its utilization by the body for growth, repair, and maintenance of health. A balanced diet provides the essential nutrients—carbohydrates, proteins, fats, vitamins, minerals, and water—that support bodily functions and promote optimal well-being.

Key Components of a Healthy Diet:

❖ Macronutrients: Carbohydrates, proteins, and fats are macronutrients that provide energy and serve as building blocks for various bodily tissues. A balanced diet includes a mix of these macronutrients, with an emphasis on whole, minimally processed sources.

❖ Micronutrients: Vitamins and minerals are micronutrients that play crucial roles in metabolism, immune function, and overall health. Consuming a diverse range of fruits, vegetables, whole grains, nuts, and seeds ensures an adequate intake of micronutrients.

❖ Hydration: Water is essential for hydration, nutrient transport, temperature regulation, and waste removal within the body. Staying adequately hydrated is vital for overall health and can support weight loss by promoting satiety and preventing overeating.

❖ Dietary Patterns: Various dietary patterns, such as the Mediterranean diet, DASH (Dietary Approaches to Stop Hypertension) diet, and plant-based diet, have been associated with numerous health benefits, including weight loss and reduced risk of chronic diseases. These patterns prioritize whole, nutrient-rich foods while minimizing processed and unhealthy options.

❖ Individualized Approach: Nutrition is highly individualized, influenced by factors such as age, gender, genetics, metabolism, activity level, and health status. Consulting with a registered dietitian or healthcare professional can help individuals develop personalized nutrition plans tailored to their specific needs and goals.

In conclusion, understanding weight loss and nutrition is essential for achieving and maintaining a healthy lifestyle. By adopting a balanced diet, engaging in regular physical activity, and making sustainable behavior and lifestyle changes, individuals can embark on a journey towards improved health, vitality, and well-being. With knowledge, dedication, and commitment, the path to weight loss and optimal nutrition becomes an empowering and fulfilling endeavor.

ESSENTIAL KITCHEN TOOLS

When embarking on a weight loss journey, having the right kitchen tools can make meal preparation easier, more efficient, and ultimately more enjoyable. Here are some essential kitchen tools for those following a weight loss diet:

1. Food Scale: Portion control is crucial for managing calorie intake. A food scale allows you to accurately measure ingredients and portion sizes, helping you stay within your calorie goals.

2. Measuring Cups and Spoons: Alongside a food scale, measuring cups and spoons are essential for precise measurement of ingredients, particularly when following recipes or portioning out servings.

3. Blender or Food Processor: A blender or food processor is versatile for creating smoothies, soups, sauces, and dips using whole, nutrient-rich ingredients. These appliances make it easy to incorporate fruits, vegetables, and other wholesome foods into your diet.

4. Vegetable Spiralizer: Swap traditional pasta for vegetable noodles made with a spiralizer. This tool allows you to create noodles from vegetables like zucchini, carrots, or sweet potatoes, providing a lower-calorie alternative to pasta.

5. Steamer Basket: Steaming vegetables is a healthy cooking method that preserves nutrients while keeping calories low. A steamer basket can be used to steam a variety of vegetables quickly and easily.

6. Non-Stick Cookware: Invest in high-quality non-stick pots and pans to minimize the need for added fats and oils during cooking. This helps reduce calorie intake without sacrificing flavor.

7. Grill Pan or Panini Press: Grilling or pressing foods can impart delicious flavor without the need for excessive oils or fats. A grill pan or Panini press allows you to cook lean proteins, vegetables, and even fruit with minimal added calories.

8. Salad Spinner: Eating salads is a great way to increase vegetable intake and promote weight loss. A salad spinner makes it easy to wash and dry leafy greens, ensuring they are crisp and ready to enjoy.

9. Air Fryer: An air fryer uses hot air circulation to cook food, producing crispy results with little to no oil. It's an excellent tool for preparing healthier versions of traditionally fried foods, such as chicken wings or sweet potato fries.

10. Storage Containers: Having a variety of storage containers in different sizes makes meal prep and portion control more manageable. Use these containers to store prepped ingredients, leftovers, and portioned meals for easy grab-and-go options.

11. Herb Mill or Herb Scissors: Fresh herbs add flavor to dishes without extra calories. A herb mill or herb scissors makes it easy to chop fresh herbs finely, enhancing the taste of your meals.

12. Water Bottle: Staying hydrated is essential for weight loss and overall health. Keep a reusable water bottle on hand to encourage regular hydration throughout the day.

FOOD TO AVOID AND TO INCLUDE

When following a weight loss diet, it's essential to focus on nutrient-dense foods that support satiety, provide essential nutrients, and promote overall health. Equally important is avoiding or limiting foods that are high in added sugars, unhealthy fats, and empty calories. Here are some foods to include and avoid on a weight loss diet:

Foods to Include:

1. Lean Proteins: Incorporate lean protein sources such as chicken breast, turkey, fish, tofu, tempeh, legumes, and low-fat dairy products. Protein helps you feel full and satisfied, making it easier to manage hunger and reduce overall calorie intake.

2. Fruits and Vegetables: Load up on a variety of colorful fruits and vegetables, which are rich in vitamins, minerals, fiber, and antioxidants. Aim to fill half of your plate with non-starchy vegetables and include fruits as a nutritious snack or dessert option.

3. Whole Grains: Choose whole grains such as quinoa, brown rice, oats, barley, and whole wheat bread and pasta. Whole grains provide fiber, which aids in digestion, promotes fullness, and helps regulate blood sugar levels.

4. Healthy Fats: Incorporate sources of healthy fats, such as avocados, nuts, seeds, olive oil, and fatty fish like salmon and mackerel. These fats are heart-healthy and help keep you feeling satisfied between meals.

5. Legumes and Beans: Beans, lentils, chickpeas, and other legumes are excellent sources of plant-based protein, fiber, and complex carbohydrates. They help stabilize blood sugar levels and promote feelings of fullness.

6. Low-Fat Dairy: Choose low-fat or non-fat dairy products such as Greek yogurt, skim milk, and cottage cheese. These dairy options provide calcium, protein, and other essential nutrients without excess calories and saturated fat.

7. Eggs: Eggs are a nutrient-dense food rich in protein and essential vitamins and minerals. They can be enjoyed in various ways, including boiled, scrambled, or poached, and make a satisfying and versatile addition to meals.

8. Herbs, Spices, and Flavorings: Use herbs, spices, citrus zest, vinegar, and other flavorings to add depth and complexity to your meals without extra calories. Experiment with different seasonings to enhance the taste of your dishes.

<u>Foods to Avoid or Limit:</u>

1. Processed Foods: Minimize consumption of processed and packaged foods high in added sugars, unhealthy fats, sodium, and preservatives. These include sugary snacks, chips, cookies, pastries, and processed meats.

2. Sugary Beverages: Avoid sugary drinks such as soda, fruit juice, energy drinks, and sweetened coffee beverages, which can contribute to excess calorie intake without providing essential nutrients.

3. Refined Carbohydrates: Limit intake of refined carbohydrates such as white bread, white rice, pasta, and sugary cereals. Instead, opt for whole grain alternatives that provide more fiber and nutrients.

4. Fried Foods: Steer clear of fried foods that are high in unhealthy fats and calories, such as French fries, fried chicken, and battered snacks. Choose healthier cooking methods such as baking, grilling, or steaming.

5. High-Calorie Snacks: Avoid calorie-dense snacks such as candy bars, chips, and sugary granola bars, which can lead to overconsumption of calories. Instead, opt for nutrient-rich snacks like fresh fruit, vegetables with hummus, or Greek yogurt.

6. Sugary Treats and Desserts: Limit intake of sugary treats and desserts such as cakes, cookies, ice cream, and candy, which are high in added sugars and empty calories. Enjoy these foods occasionally in moderation.

7. Alcohol: Limit alcohol consumption, as it provides empty calories and can interfere with weight loss goals. Choose lower-calorie options such as light beer or wine in moderation, and be mindful of portion sizes.

By focusing on nutrient-dense foods and minimizing or avoiding processed, high-calorie options, you can support your weight loss efforts while nourishing your body with essential nutrients. Remember to practice portion control, stay hydrated, and maintain a balanced diet to achieve long-term success in reaching your weight loss goals.

GROCERY SHOPPING GUIDE

Creating a grocery shopping guide tailored to a weight loss diet involves selecting nutrient-dense foods that support satiety, provide essential nutrients, and promote overall health. Here's a comprehensive grocery shopping guide to help you make healthier choices and stay on track with your weight loss goals:

Produce Section:
- Leafy greens (spinach, kale, arugula, lettuce)
- Cruciferous vegetables (broccoli, cauliflower, Brussels sprouts)
- Colorful vegetables (bell peppers, carrots, tomatoes, cucumbers)
- Berries (strawberries, blueberries, raspberries)
- Citrus fruits (oranges, lemons, limes)
- Avocados
- Apples and pears
- Bananas
- Garlic and onions
- Fresh herbs (parsley, cilantro, basil)

Deli and Meat Department:
- Skinless poultry (chicken breast, turkey breast)
- Lean cuts of beef (sirloin, tenderloin)
- Lean cuts of pork (loin, tenderloin)
- Fish (salmon, tuna, trout, cod)
- Shellfish (shrimp, scallops)
- Lean deli meats (turkey, chicken)
- Eggs
- Tofu or tempeh (for plant-based protein options)

Dairy and Alternatives:
- Low-fat or non-fat Greek yogurt
- Skim or low-fat milk
- Cottage cheese
- Reduced-fat cheese
- Unsweetened almond milk, soy milk, or other plant-based milk alternatives
- Reduced-fat sour cream

Grains and Cereals:
- Whole grain bread (whole wheat, multigrain)
- Whole grain pasta (whole wheat, brown rice)
- Quinoa
- Brown rice
- Oats (rolled oats, steel-cut oats)
- Barley
- Whole grain cereal with minimal added sugars
- Whole grain tortillas or wraps

Legumes and Beans:
- Lentils
- Black beans
- Chickpeas
- Kidney beans
- Cannellini beans
- Pinto beans

Nuts, Seeds, and Nut Butters:
- Almonds
- Walnuts
- Pistachios
- Chia seeds
- Flaxseeds
- Hemp seeds
- Natural peanut butter or almond butter (without added sugars or hydrogenated oils)

Frozen Foods:
- Frozen fruits (berries, mango chunks, pineapple)
- Frozen vegetables (broccoli, cauliflower, spinach)

- Frozen pre-portioned meals with lean protein and vegetables (check labels for sodium and added sugars)

Canned Goods:
- Canned tuna or salmon (in water)
- Canned beans (black beans, chickpeas, kidney beans)
- Canned tomatoes (diced, crushed, or whole)
- Low-sodium chicken or vegetable broth
- Canned vegetables (corn, green beans, peas)

Condiments and Flavorings:
- Olive oil or avocado oil
- Balsamic vinegar
- Dijon mustard
- Low-sodium soy sauce or tamari
- Hot sauce or salsa (without added sugars)
- Herbs and spices (oregano, basil, cumin, paprika, cinnamon)

- Low-sodium broth or stock (chicken, vegetable)

Snacks:
- Fresh fruit (apples, bananas, oranges)
- Baby carrots or sliced cucumbers with hummus
- Air-popped popcorn
- Rice cakes with almond butter
- Low-fat string cheese or cheese sticks
- Greek yogurt with berries
- Raw nuts or seeds (portioned to avoid overeating)

Beverages:
- Water (sparkling or still)
- Herbal tea (unsweetened)
- Coffee (black or with a splash of milk)
- Unsweetened almond milk, soy milk, or other plant-based milk alternatives
- Sparkling water (flavored or plain)

When grocery shopping for weight loss, focus on filling your cart with whole, minimally processed foods that are rich in nutrients and low in added sugars, unhealthy fats, and sodium. Planning ahead, making a shopping list, and sticking to the perimeter of the grocery store (where fresh produce, lean proteins, and dairy products are typically located) can help you make healthier choices and avoid impulse purchases. Remember to read food labels and ingredient lists to make informed decisions about the foods you buy. With a well-stocked kitchen and a commitment to healthier eating habits, you'll be well-equipped to achieve your weight loss goals and improve your overall well-being.

BREAKFAST RECIPES

Greek Yogurt Parfait

Cooking Time: None | **Prep Time**: 5 minutes | **Total Time**: 5 minutes | **Serving Size**: 1 Serving

Ingredients:

- 150g Plain Greek Yogurt (2% fat)
- 100g Mixed berries (fresh or frozen)
- 50g Unsweetened granola
- 1/4 tsp Ground cinnamon (optional)

Directions:

1. Prepare the Yogurt: If desired, stir a small amount of water or unsweetened almond milk into the yogurt to achieve a thinner consistency. You can also leave it thick for a more filling option.
2. Assemble the Parfait: In a serving glass or jar, layer 1/2 of the yogurt on the bottom.
3. Add the Fruit: Top the yogurt with 1/2 of the mixed berries.
4. Sprinkle the Granola: Evenly distribute 1/2 of the granola over the fruit layer.
5. Repeat Layers: Add another layer of yogurt, another layer of fruit, and the remaining granola on top.
6. **Season (Optional): Sprinkle with a pinch of ground cinnamon for added flavor and warmth.
7. Serve Immediately: Enjoy your parfait fresh for the best texture and flavor.

Nutritional Information per serving: Calories: 250, Fat: 5g, Carbs: 25g, Fiber: 5g, Protein: 20g

Tips:

- Use low-fat or fat-free Greek yogurt for even lower calorie content.
- Sweeten the yogurt naturally with a squeeze of fresh lemon juice or a sprinkle of stevia powder instead of sugar.
- Substitute the mixed berries with other low-calorie fruits like chopped apple, mango, or papaya.
- Add a drizzle of chia seeds or chopped nuts for extra protein and crunch.
- Prepare parfaits in advance and store them in airtight containers in the refrigerator for up to 2 days.

Vegetable Omelette

Prep Time: 5 minutes | **Cooking Time**: 10 minutes | **Total Time**: 15 minutes | **Servings**: 1

Ingredients:

- 2 large eggs
- 1 tablespoon low-fat milk (optional)
- 1/2 cup chopped mixed vegetables (such as onions, bell peppers, mushrooms, spinach)
- 1/4 cup chopped tomato
- 1/4 cup shredded low-fat cheddar cheese
- Salt and pepper to taste

Directions:

1. Whisk together the eggs and milk (if using) in a bowl. Season with salt and pepper.
2. Heat a non-stick pan over medium heat. Spray with cooking spray.
3. Add the chopped vegetables and cook until softened, about 3-5 minutes.
4. Pour the egg mixture into the pan and tilt the pan to spread the eggs evenly.
5. Let the omelette cook for a few minutes until the bottom is set.
6. Sprinkle the cheese and tomato over one half of the omelette.
7. Fold the other half of the omelette over the filling.
8. Cook for another minute or two until the cheese is melted and the omelette is cooked through.
9. Slide the omelette onto a plate and enjoy!

Nutritional Information per serving: Calories: 250, Fat: 10g, Carbs: 7g, Protein: 20g, Fiber: 3g, Sodium: 150mg

Tips:

- For a lighter option, use egg whites only.
- Add additional vegetables to your liking, such as broccoli, zucchini, or carrots.
- Use spices like oregano, basil, or cumin to add flavor.
- Serve with a side of whole-wheat toast or fruit for a complete meal.

Quinoa Breakfast Bowl

Prep Time: 5 minutes | **Cooking Time**: 15 minutes | **Total Time**: 20 minutes | **Serving Size**: 1

Ingredients:

- 1/2 cup dry quinoa, rinsed
- 1 cup water or vegetable broth
- 1/4 cup chopped spinach
- 1/4 cup crumbled feta cheese
- 1/4 cup chopped avocado
- 1/4 cup cherry tomatoes, halved
- 1/2 teaspoon olive oil
- Salt and pepper to taste

Directions:

1. In a pot, combine quinoa and water or broth. Bring to a boil, then reduce heat, cover, and simmer for 15 minutes, or until quinoa is fluffy and cooked through.

2. While the quinoa is cooking, prepare the other ingredients.

3. Once the quinoa is cooked, fluff it with a fork and spread it evenly in a bowl.

4. Top with the spinach, feta cheese, avocado, tomatoes, and olive oil.

5. Season with salt and pepper to taste.

Nutritional Information: Calories: 350, Protein: 18g, Fiber: 8g, Fat: 8g, Carbs: 35g

Tips:

- For a heartier bowl, you can add a cooked egg (poached, scrambled, or hard-boiled) or lean protein like grilled chicken or fish.
- You can also add a sprinkle of spices like cumin, chili powder, or paprika for added flavor.
- If you don't have cherry tomatoes, you can use other vegetables like chopped bell peppers, cucumbers, or carrots.
- To make this bowl vegan, use a plant-based milk or broth and omit the feta cheese.

Whole Grain Toast with Avocado and Egg

Prep Time: 5 minutes | **Cooking Time**: 10 minutes | **Total Time**: 15 minutes | **Servings**: 1

Ingredients:

- 1 slice whole grain bread (sourdough, Ezekiel, pumpernickel, etc.)
- 1/2 medium avocado, ripe
- 1 large egg
- 1 tablespoon milk (optional, for scrambled eggs)
- Salt and pepper to taste
- optional toppings:
- Hot sauce
- Red pepper flakes
- Sliced cherry tomatoes
- Chopped spinach

Directions:

1. Toast the bread: Using a toaster or pan, toast your bread to your desired level of crispness.
2. Prepare the avocado: Mash the avocado with a fork in a small bowl. Season with a pinch of salt and pepper.
3. Cook the egg: Choose your preferred cooking method:
   - Scrambled: In a small pan heated with a bit of olive oil, whisk together the egg and milk (if using). Scramble until cooked through.
   - Fried: Heat a small amount of oil in a pan. Crack the egg and fry until the white is set and the yolk is cooked to your liking.
   - Poached: Bring a pot of water to a simmer. Crack the egg into a small bowl and gently slip it into the simmering water. Cook for 3-4 minutes until the whites are set and the yolk is runny.
4. Assemble: Spread the mashed avocado on the toasted bread. Top with the cooked egg. Season with additional salt and pepper if desired.
5. Serve immediately and enjoy!

Nutritional Information Per serving: Calories: 331, Fat: 20g (5g saturated), Carbohydrates: 21g (6g fiber), Protein: 18g

Tips:

- Use a smaller slice of bread to control overall calorie intake.
- Opt for a low-fat cooking method for the egg, such as poaching or scrambling with minimal oil.
- Limit additional toppings or choose low-calorie options like hot sauce or red pepper flakes.
- Pair this toast with a side of fruit or vegetables for added vitamins and fiber.

Chia Seed Pudding

Cooking Time: 0 minutes | **Prep Time**: 5 minutes | **Total Time**: 12-18 hours | **Serving Size**: 1

Ingredients:

- 1/4 cup chia seeds
- 1 cup unsweetened almond milk
- 1/4 teaspoon vanilla extract (optional)
- Pinch of cinnamon (optional)

Directions:

1. Combine ingredients: In a small bowl or jar, whisk together the chia seeds, almond milk, vanilla extract (if using), and cinnamon (if using). Ensure everything is well combined.

2. Soak overnight: Cover the bowl or jar and refrigerate for at least 12 hours, or preferably overnight. The chia seeds will absorb the liquid and expand, creating a thick pudding-like consistency.

3. Serve: In the morning, stir the pudding well. You can enjoy it plain or add toppings like fresh fruit, chopped nuts, or a sprinkle of unsweetened cocoa powder.

Nutritional Information: Calories: 230, Fat: 12g (2g saturated), Carbohydrates: 14g (4g fiber), Protein: 5g, Sugar: 1g

Tips:

- For a thicker pudding, use less liquid. For a thinner pudding, use more liquid.
- You can use different types of milk, such as coconut milk, oat milk, or cow's milk. Be mindful of the calorie and sugar content of different options.
- Experiment with different spices and flavorings, such as nutmeg, ginger, or a splash of lemon juice.
- Feel free to add a teaspoon of stevia or monk fruit sweetener for a touch of sweetness.
- This pudding is best enjoyed fresh, but it can be stored in the refrigerator for up to 3 days.

Smoothie Bowl

Cooking Time: 0 minutes | **Prep Time**: 5 minutes | **Total Time**: 5 minutes | **Serving Size**: 1 bowl

Ingredients:

- 1 cup unsweetened almond milk
- 1/2 cup frozen spinach
- 1/2 frozen banana
- 1/4 cup rolled oats
- 1 scoop protein powder (unflavored or vanilla)
- 1/4 cup blueberries
- 1/4 cup chopped strawberries

Optional Toppings:

- Chia seeds
- Hemp seeds
- Sliced almonds
- Coconut flakes
- Unsweetened shredded coconut
- Cacao nibs

Directions:

1. Prep: Wash and chop the strawberries. If using fresh spinach, wash and roughly chop it.

2. Blend: Combine all ingredients except the blueberries and strawberries in a blender and blend until smooth.

3. Assemble: Pour the smoothie into a bowl. Top with the blueberries, strawberries, and any other desired toppings (see optional below).

4. Enjoy!

Nutritional Information: Calories: 320, Protein: 12g, Carbs: 35g, Fiber: 8g, Fat: 10g (5g healthy fats)

Tips:

- If using fresh spinach, make sure it's tightly packed in the measuring cup.
- For a thicker consistency, add more frozen banana or ice cubes.
- Substitute the protein powder with another scoop of rolled oats or chia seeds for a less protein-rich bowl.
- Adjust the sweetness to your preference by adding a little bit of honey or maple syrup.
- This smoothie bowl is best enjoyed immediately. However, it can be stored in an airtight container in the freezer for up to 2 days.

Egg Muffins

Prep Time: 10 minutes | **Cooking Time**: 15-20 minutes | **Total Time**: 30 minutes | **Servings**: 6 muffins

Ingredients:

- 6 eggs
- 1/4 cup unsweetened almond milk
- 1/4 cup chopped spinach
- 1/4 cup chopped bell pepper
- 1/4 cup chopped mushrooms
- 1/4 cup crumbled feta cheese
- 1/4 teaspoon dried oregano
- 1/4 teaspoon garlic powder
- Salt and pepper to taste

Directions:

1. Preheat oven to 350°F (175°C). Grease a 6-cup muffin tin with cooking spray or non-stick baking spray.

2. In a large bowl, whisk together eggs and almond milk.

3. Stir in spinach, bell pepper, mushrooms, feta cheese, oregano, garlic powder, salt, and pepper.

4. Divide the mixture evenly between the prepared muffin cups.

5. Bake for 15-20 minutes, or until eggs are set and cooked through.

6. Let cool slightly before removing from the muffin tin.

Nutritional Information per muffin: Calories: 120, Fat: 8g, Carbs: 2g, Protein: 10g, Fiber: 1g

Tips:

- For a spicier option, add a pinch of red pepper flakes.
- Substitute other vegetables like broccoli, onions, or tomatoes.
- Use different cheeses like cheddar, mozzarella, or cottage cheese.
- Add cooked lean protein like turkey sausage or crumbled chicken breast for extra protein.
- Store leftover muffins in an airtight container in the refrigerator for up to 3 days.
- Reheat in the microwave or oven for a quick and easy breakfast or snack.

Cottage Cheese Pancakes

Prep Time: 5 minutes | **Cooking Time**: 10-15 minutes | **Total Time**: 20-25 minutes | **Serving Size**: 2-3 pancakes

Ingredients:

- 1/2 cup low-fat cottage cheese
- 1/4 cup unsweetened applesauce
- 1 egg
- 1/4 cup rolled oats
- 1/4 teaspoon baking powder
- Pinch of salt
- Optional toppings: fresh fruit, Greek yogurt, sugar-free syrup

Directions:

1. In a blender or food processor, combine cottage cheese, applesauce, egg, rolled oats, baking powder, and salt. Blend until smooth and well combined.

2. Heat a lightly greased non-stick pan or griddle over medium heat.

3. Pour about 1/4 cup of batter per pancake onto the pan. Cook for 2-3 minutes per side, or until golden brown and cooked through.

4. Flip the pancakes carefully using a spatula.

5. Repeat steps 3 and 4 with remaining batter.

6. Serve immediately with your desired toppings.

Nutritional Information per pancake: Calories: 150-180, Protein: 15-20g, Carbs: 15-20g, Fat: 5-7g, Fiber: 2-3g

Tips:

- For a smoother texture, blend the cottage cheese until very creamy before adding the other ingredients.
- If the batter seems too thick, add a tablespoon of milk or water to thin it out.
- Don't overcook the pancakes, as they will become dry.
- For a thicker pancake, use slightly more batter per pancake.
- Top with fresh fruit for added sweetness and vitamins.
- You can use spices like cinnamon or nutmeg for additional flavor.

Overnight Oats

Prep Time: 5 minutes | **Cooking Time**: None | **Total Time**: 5 minutes | **Serving Size**: 1

Ingredients:

- 1/2 cup rolled oats (not quick oats)
- 1 cup unsweetened almond milk (or other low-fat milk)
- 1/4 cup plain Greek yogurt (optional, for added protein)
- 1 tablespoon chia seeds
- 1/2 teaspoon ground cinnamon
- Pinch of salt

Directions:

1. In a sealable container, combine the rolled oats, almond milk, yogurt (if using), chia seeds, cinnamon, and salt. Stir well to ensure everything is mixed evenly.

2. Cover the container tightly and refrigerate for at least 8 hours, ideally overnight.

3. In the morning, stir the oats again. The oats will have absorbed the liquid and become soft and creamy.

4. Enjoy as is, or top with fresh fruit (berries, sliced apple, etc.) for additional sweetness and nutrients.

Nutritional Information: Calories: 240, Fat: 4g, Carbohydrates: 40g, Fiber: 5g, Protein: 6g, Sugar: 5g

Tips:

- Use rolled oats for optimal texture and nutrition. Quick oats tend to become mushy.
- Adjust the liquid amount based on desired consistency. Add more for a creamier texture, or less for a thicker oatmeal.
- For extra protein, consider adding a scoop of protein powder.
- Avoid adding high-calorie ingredients like sugary syrups, chocolate chips, or excessive nut butters.
- Experiment with different spices like nutmeg, ginger, or cardamom for flavor variations.
- This recipe is a base, feel free to customize it with your favorite low-calorie fruits, nuts, or seeds.

Egg and Veggie Breakfast Burrito

Cooking Time: 15 minutes | **Prep Time**: 10 minutes | **Total Time**: 25 minutes | **Servings**: 1

Ingredients:

- 1 large whole wheat tortilla (60g)
- 2 large eggs (120g)
- 1/2 cup chopped mixed vegetables (bell pepper, onion, spinach, mushrooms - choose your favorites!) (50g)
- 1/4 cup black beans, rinsed and drained (50g)
- 1 tablespoon salsa (20g)
- 1/4 avocado, sliced (30g)
- Salt and pepper to taste

Directions:

1. Prep your veggies: Wash and chop your chosen vegetables into bite-sized pieces.

2. Cook the eggs: In a non-stick pan, heat a small amount of cooking spray over medium heat. Scramble the eggs until cooked through, season with salt and pepper.

3. Sauté the veggies: In the same pan used for the eggs, add a drizzle of cooking spray and saute the chopped vegetables until tender-crisp, about 5 minutes. Season with salt and pepper.

4. Assemble the burrito: Lay out your tortilla on a plate. Spread with a thin layer of salsa. Top with half of the scrambled eggs, then layer on the black beans, cooked vegetables, and avocado slices.

5. Roll and enjoy: Carefully fold the bottom of the tortilla over the filling, then fold in the sides. Roll up tightly and enjoy!

Nutritional Information: Calories: 350, Fat: 10g, Carbohydrates: 30g, Fiber: 5g, Protein: 20g

Tips:

- For added protein, you can crumble in 1/4 cup cooked lean ground turkey or chicken sausage with the vegetables.
- For a spicy kick, add a few dashes of your favorite hot sauce.
- Use low-sodium black beans and salsa to keep your sodium intake in check.
- Toast your tortilla in a dry pan for a few seconds before assembly for extra flavor and texture.
- Serve with a side of fruit or yogurt for a complete and balanced breakfast.

Zucchini Fritters

Prep Time: 15 minutes | **Cook Time**: 20 minutes | **Total Time**: 35 minutes | **Servings**: 4

Ingredients:

- 2 medium zucchinis, grated
- 1/4 cup chopped onion
- 1/4 cup chopped fresh herbs (dill, parsley, or cilantro)
- 1 egg
- 1/4 cup whole wheat flour
- 1/4 cup chickpea flour
- 1 teaspoon baking powder
- 1/4 teaspoon garlic powder
- Pinch of salt and pepper
- Cooking spray

Directions:

1. Grate the zucchini: Grate the zucchini using a box grater. Place the grated zucchini in a colander and sprinkle with 1/2 teaspoon of salt. Let it sit for 10 minutes to release excess moisture. Press the zucchini with a paper towel to remove as much liquid as possible.
2. Combine dry ingredients: In a bowl, whisk together the whole wheat flour, chickpea flour, baking powder, garlic powder, salt, and pepper.
3. Mix the batter: In a separate bowl, whisk together the egg. Add the zucchini, onion, and herbs to the egg mixture, then stir in the dry ingredients until just combined.
4. Cook the fritters: Heat a non-stick pan or griddle over medium heat and spray with cooking spray. Spoon about 1/4 cup of batter per fritter into the pan. Cook for 3-4 minutes per side, or until golden brown and cooked through.
5. Serve: Enjoy your zucchini fritters warm with a side of Greek yogurt or a low-fat dipping sauce.

Nutritional Information per Serving: Calories: 150, Fat: 5g, Carbohydrates: 15g (including 4g fiber), Protein: 5g, Sodium: 200mg

Tips:

- You can add a grated carrot or apple to the batter for additional sweetness and crunch.
- Use a non-stick pan or griddle to prevent sticking.
- Don't overcook the fritters, or they will become dry and tough.
- Make sure the zucchini is well-drained to prevent the fritters from being soggy.
- For a lighter option, bake the fritters in a preheated oven at 400°F for 15-20 minutes, flipping halfway through.

Chia Pudding with Almond Milk and Fruits

Cooking Time: None | **Prep Time**: 5 minutes | **Total Time**: 4 hours | **Serving Size**: 1

Ingredients:

- 3/4 cup unsweetened almond milk
- 1/4 cup chia seeds
- 1/2 teaspoon vanilla extract
- 1/4 teaspoon ground cinnamon (optional)
- 1/4 cup mixed berries (fresh or frozen)
- 1/4 cup sliced banana

Directions:

1. In a jar or container with a lid, combine the almond milk, chia seeds, vanilla extract, and cinnamon (if using). Stir well to combine.

2. Cover the jar and refrigerate for at least 4 hours, or overnight. The chia seeds will absorb the liquid and thicken into a pudding-like consistency.

3. In the morning, top the chia pudding with the mixed berries and sliced banana. Enjoy!

Nutritional Information per serving: Calories: 240, Fat: 9g, Carbohydrates: 24g, Fiber: 11g, Protein: 5g, Sugar: 8g (depending on the sweetness of the fruit)

Tips:

- You can use any type of milk you like, but almond milk is lower in calories and fat than full-fat dairy milk.
- For a thicker pudding, use less liquid or soak for longer. For a thinner pudding, use more liquid or soak for less time.
- You can add other toppings to your chia pudding, such as chopped nuts, shredded coconut, or a drizzle of honey or maple syrup.
- Make sure to use ripe bananas for the best flavor.
- If you don't have fresh berries, you can use frozen berries that have been thawed.
- You can store leftover chia pudding in the refrigerator for up to 3 days.

Egg White Veggie Scramble

Prep Time: 5 minutes | **Cooking Time**: 10 minutes | **Total Time**: 15 minutes | **Serving Size**: 1

Ingredients:

- 4 egg whites
- 1/2 cup chopped vegetables (bell peppers, onions, mushrooms, spinach, etc.)
- 1/4 cup chopped cherry tomatoes
- 1/4 cup chopped fresh herbs (optional but recommended for flavor)
- 1 tablespoon olive oil
- Salt and pepper to taste
- Optional: 1/4 teaspoon low-sodium soy sauce or hot sauce for added flavor

Directions:

1. Prep the vegetables: Wash and chop all your vegetables. If using tomatoes, halve them if desired. Preheat a non-stick pan over medium heat.

2. Cook the vegetables: Add the olive oil to the pan and heat it up. Sauté the onions and peppers for 2-3 minutes until softened. Stir in the remaining vegetables (except tomatoes) and cook for another 3-4 minutes until tender-crisp.

3. Scramble the egg whites: In a separate bowl, whisk the egg whites with salt and pepper. Pour the egg whites into the pan with the vegetables, spreading them evenly.

4. Cook the eggs: Let the eggs cook undisturbed for about 1 minute, then start gently scrambling them with a spatula until cooked through.

5. Add finishing touches: Stir in the cherry tomatoes and fresh herbs (if using). Cook for another minute until the tomatoes are warmed through. Season with additional salt and pepper to taste.

6. Serve: Enjoy your egg white veggie scramble immediately.

Nutritional Information per serving: Calories: 250, Protein: 25g, Fat: 5g, Carbohydrates: 5g, Fiber: 2g

Tips:

- Use a nonstick pan to prevent sticking.
- Adjust the cooking time of the vegetables depending on your desired texture.
- Experiment with different types of vegetables to keep things interesting.
- To make it even more filling, add a crumbled piece of low-fat cheese on top.
- This recipe can easily be doubled or tripled to feed more people.

Cauliflower Hash Browns

Prep Time: 10 minutes | **Cooking Time**: 15 minutes | **Total Time**: 25 minutes | **Serving Size**: 1

Ingredients:

- 1 head cauliflower, grated or pulsed in a food processor
- 1 egg
- 1/4 cup chopped onion
- 1/4 teaspoon garlic powder
- 1/4 teaspoon dried oregano
- Salt and pepper to taste

Directions:

1. Prepare the cauliflower: Grate the cauliflower by hand or pulse it in a food processor until it resembles rice. Place the grated cauliflower in a clean kitchen towel and squeeze out as much excess moisture as possible. This is crucial for crispy hash browns.
2. Combine the ingredients: In a large bowl, whisk together the egg, onion, garlic powder, oregano, salt, and pepper. Add the squeezed cauliflower and mix well to combine.
3. Cook the hash browns: Heat a non-stick pan over medium heat. Spray with cooking spray or brush with a thin layer of oil. Form the cauliflower mixture into small patties (about 3 inches in diameter). Cook for 3-4 minutes per side, or until golden brown and crispy.
4. Serve: Enjoy your cauliflower hash browns hot with your favorite breakfast toppings, such as avocado, salsa, or a fried egg.

Nutritional Information: Calories: 120, Fat: 3g, Carbs: 8g (5g net carbs), Fiber: 3g, Protein: 5g

Tips:

- For extra flavor, you can add a pinch of cayenne pepper or your favorite herbs and spices.
- If you don't have a food processor, you can finely grate the cauliflower using a box grater.
- If your hash browns are not sticking together, add another egg or a tablespoon of almond flour.
- To make them ahead of time, cook the hash browns as directed and then store them in an airtight container in the refrigerator for up to 3 days. Reheat in a pan or toaster oven until warmed through.

Spinach and Feta Breakfast Wrap

Prep Time: 5 minutes | **Cooking Time**: 10 minutes | **Total Time**: 15 minutes | **Serving Size**: 1 wrap

Ingredients:

- 1 large whole-wheat tortilla (60g)
- 2 large eggs (120g)
- 1/2 cup fresh baby spinach (50g)
- 1/4 cup crumbled feta cheese (40g)
- 1/4 teaspoon olive oil
- Salt and black pepper to taste

Directions:

1. Prep: Wash and dry the spinach. Crumble the feta cheese. Whisk the eggs in a bowl with salt and pepper. Preheat a non-stick pan over medium heat.

2. Cook the Eggs: Heat the olive oil in the pan. Pour in the whisked eggs and scramble until cooked through, about 2-3 minutes.

3. Wilting the Spinach: Add the spinach to the cooked eggs and cook for another minute, stirring occasionally, until the spinach is wilted.

4. Assemble the Wrap: Lay the tortilla out on a plate. Spread the scrambled egg and spinach mixture evenly over one half of the tortilla. Sprinkle with feta cheese.

5. Wrap it Up: Fold the empty half of the tortilla over the filling, enclosing it completely. You can fold it like a burrito or envelope style.

6. Optional Toast: If desired, toast the wrap in a dry pan over medium heat for a few seconds on each side for a crispier texture.

7. Enjoy! Serve your wrap immediately while hot.

Nutritional Information per serving: Calories: 280, Fat: 8g, Carbs: 28g, Fiber: 4g, Protein: 16g, Sodium: 300mg (depending on feta brand)

Tips:

- For a vegan option, use tofu scramble instead of eggs.
- Add a touch of hot sauce or salsa for extra flavor.
- Use reduced-fat feta cheese to further reduce calories and fat.
- Pack the leftover wrap for a healthy on-the-go breakfast.

Berry Protein Pancakes

Prep Time: 5 minutes | **Cooking Time**: 10 minutes | **Total Time**: 15 minutes | **Serving Size**: 2 pancakes

Ingredients:

- 1/2 cup rolled oats (40g)
- 1 scoop (25g) unflavored or vanilla protein powder
- 1/2 teaspoon baking powder
- 1/4 teaspoon cinnamon
- 1/4 cup unsweetened almond milk
- 1 egg white
- 1/4 cup fresh or frozen berries

Directions:

1. In a blender, grind the rolled oats into a fine flour.

2. Add the protein powder, baking powder, and cinnamon to the blender and blend until combined.

3. In a separate bowl, whisk together the almond milk and egg white.

4. Pour the wet ingredients into the dry ingredients and mix until just combined. Do not over mix.

5. Heat a non-stick pan over medium heat. Lightly spray with cooking spray.

6. Pour 1/4 cup of batter onto the pan for each pancake.

7. Cook for 2-3 minutes per side, or until golden brown and cooked through.

8. Top with your favorite berries and enjoy!

Nutritional Information per serving: Calories: 250, Fat: 5g, Carbohydrates: 25g, Fiber: 5g, Protein: 20g, Sugar: 5g

Tips:

- For a sweeter pancake, you can add a few drops of stevia or a teaspoon of natural maple syrup to the batter.
- If the batter is too thick, you can add a splash more almond milk to thin it out.
- You can use any type of protein powder you like, but unflavored or vanilla will work best in this recipe.
- Serve with a dollop of Greek yogurt or cottage cheese for an extra protein boost.
- Feel free to experiment with different toppings, such as sliced almonds, chia seeds, or chopped nuts.

Sweet Potato Breakfast Bowl

Prep Time: 10 minutes | **Cooking Time**: 30 minutes | **Total Time**: 40 minutes | **Serving Size**: 1 bowl

Ingredients:

- 1 medium sweet potato (about 6 oz)
- 1/2 cup chopped spinach
- 1/4 cup chopped bell pepper (any color)
- 1/4 cup chopped onion
- 1/4 cup crumbled low-fat feta cheese
- 1 egg
- 1/4 teaspoon ground cumin
- 1/4 teaspoon chili powder
- Salt and pepper to taste
- Non-stick cooking spray

Directions:

1. Prepare the sweet potato: Wash and pierce the sweet potato with a fork several times. Microwave on high for 5-7 minutes, flipping halfway through, until tender. While the potato cooks, prepare the other ingredients.
2. Sauté the vegetables: Heat non-stick cooking spray in a pan over medium heat. Add the onion and bell pepper and cook for 3-4 minutes, until softened. Add the spinach and cook until wilted.
3. Cook the egg: In a separate pan, spray with non-stick cooking spray and heat over medium heat. Crack the egg in and scramble until cooked through.
4. Assemble the bowl: Once the sweet potato is cooked, slice it open and scoop the flesh into a bowl. Top with the sautéed vegetables, crumbled feta cheese, scrambled egg, and sprinkle with cumin and chili powder. Season with salt and pepper to taste.

Nutritional Information per serving: Calories: 350, Fat: 5g, Saturated Fat: 1g, Carbohydrates: 45g, Fiber: 7g, Sugars: 15g, Protein: 10g

Tips:

- For a quicker preparation, you can roast the sweet potato in the oven the night before. Simply preheat the oven to 400°F (200°C), pierce the potato with a fork, and roast for 30-40 minutes, until tender.
- Add a touch of hot sauce for extra flavor and a metabolism boost.
- Substitute low-fat Greek yogurt for the feta cheese for a further protein boost.
- Top with fresh herbs like cilantro or parsley for an extra pop of flavor.
- If you prefer a warmer bowl, reheat the sweet potato for a few seconds before assembling.

Egg and Veggie Breakfast Casserole

Prep Time: 15 minutes | **Cooking Time**: 35-40 minutes | **Total Time**: 50-55 minutes | **Serving Size**: 6 slices

Ingredients:

- 1 tablespoon olive oil
- 1 medium onion, diced
- 1 red bell pepper, diced
- 1 green bell pepper, diced
- 2 cups broccoli florets
- 2 cups baby spinach, chopped
- 8 eggs
- ½ cup unsweetened almond milk
- ¼ cup chopped fresh parsley
- ½ teaspoon garlic powder
- ½ teaspoon dried oregano
- ¼ teaspoon salt
- ¼ teaspoon black pepper
- 1 cup shredded low-fat mozzarella cheese

Directions:

1. Preheat oven to 375°F (190°C). Lightly grease a 9x13 inch baking dish.
2. Heat olive oil in a large skillet over medium heat. Add onion and cook for 5 minutes, until softened. Add bell peppers and broccoli, cook for an additional 5 minutes, until slightly softened. Stir in spinach and cook until wilted. Remove from heat and set aside.
3. In a large bowl, whisk together eggs, almond milk, parsley, garlic powder, oregano, salt, and pepper.
4. Spread the veggie mixture evenly in the prepared baking dish. Pour the egg mixture over the veggies.
5. Sprinkle with mozzarella cheese.
6. Bake for 35-40 minutes, or until the eggs are set and the cheese is golden brown.
7. Let cool slightly before slicing and serving.

Nutritional Information per slice: Calories: 250, Fat: 10g, Protein: 20g, Carbs: 15g, Fiber: 2g

Tips:
- For added protein, you can stir in cooked lean chicken sausage or turkey crumbles with the veggies.
- If you prefer a creamier casserole, use ¼ cup of low-fat Greek yogurt instead of almond milk.
- Add a kick of spice with a pinch of red pepper flakes.
- For a vegetarian option, omit the parmesan cheese or use a vegetarian substitute.
- Store leftovers in an airtight container in the refrigerator for up to 3 days.
- Reheat individual slices in the microwave or oven until warmed through.

Apple Cinnamon Baked Oatmeal

Cooking Time: 35-40 minutes | **Prep Time**: 10 minutes | **Total Time**: 45-50 minutes | **Serving Size**: 1

Ingredients:

- 1/2 cup (40g) rolled oats
- 1/2 cup (120ml) unsweetened almond milk
- 1/4 cup (60ml) unsweetened applesauce
- 1 egg white
- 1/4 teaspoon ground cinnamon
- 1/8 teaspoon ground nutmeg
- 1/4 teaspoon baking powder
- Pinch of salt
- 1/2 medium apple, peeled and diced (about 1/2 cup)

Directions:

1. Preheat oven to 375°F (190°C). Lightly grease an 8x8 inch baking dish with non-stick spray.

2. In a large bowl, whisk together oats, almond milk, applesauce, egg white, cinnamon, nutmeg, baking powder, and salt.

3. Fold in the diced apples.

4. Pour the oatmeal mixture into the prepared baking dish.

5. Bake for 35-40 minutes, or until the center is set and a toothpick inserted comes out clean.

6. Let cool slightly before serving.

Nutritional Information per Serving: Calories: 300, Fat: 8g, Carbs: 40g, Fiber: 6g, Protein: 10g, Sugar: 15g

Tips:

- For added sweetness, you can sprinkle on a pinch of stevia or a couple of drops of sugar-free vanilla extract.
- Top your oatmeal with a dollop of Greek yogurt, a handful of chopped nuts, or some chia seeds for extra protein and nutrients.
- This recipe can easily be doubled or tripled to make a larger batch for meal prep.
- Feel free to experiment with different spices, such as ginger, cardamom, or cloves.
- You can also add a handful of chopped nuts or seeds for added crunch and texture.

Fruit and Nut Breakfast Bowl

Cooking Time: None | **Prep Time**: 5 minutes | **Total Time**: 5 minutes | **Serving Size**: 1 person

Ingredients:

- 1/2 cup plain Greek yogurt (unsweetened or lightly sweetened)
- 1/2 cup mixed berries (fresh or frozen)
- 1/4 cup rolled oats
- 1/4 cup chopped nuts (almonds, walnuts, pecans, etc.)
- 1/2 teaspoon chia seeds
- 1/4 teaspoon ground cinnamon (optional)

Directions:

1. In a bowl, combine the plain Greek yogurt.

2. Top with the mixed berries.

3. Sprinkle the rolled oats, chopped nuts, and chia seeds on top.

4. Dust with ground cinnamon, if desired.

5. Enjoy immediately!

Nutritional Information: Calories: 350, Fat: 10g, Carbs: 35g, Fiber: 8g, Protein: 10g, Sugar: 20g (natural sugars from fruits)

Tips:

- For a thicker consistency, use less yogurt or thicker Greek yogurt.
- For a creamier texture, blend half of the berries with the yogurt before adding them to the bowl.
- Substitute different fruits based on your preference and seasonality.
- Add a drizzle of honey, maple syrup, or agave nectar for a touch of sweetness, but be mindful of added sugar.
- Chia seeds can be soaked in the yogurt overnight for a thicker, pudding-like texture.
- Feel free to add a dash of vanilla extract or almond extract for extra flavor.
- For added protein, top with hemp seeds, pumpkin seeds, or a scoop of protein powder.
- You can pre-portion the ingredients in individual containers for a grab-and-go breakfast.

Grilled Chicken Salad

Prep Time: 10 minutes | **Cooking Time**: 15 minutes | **Total Time**: 25 minutes | **Serving Size**: 1

Ingredients:

- 1 boneless, skinless chicken breast
- 1 tablespoon olive oil
- 1/2 teaspoon salt
- 1/4 teaspoon black pepper
- 2 cups mixed greens (spinach, romaine, arugula)
- 1/2 cup cherry tomatoes, halved
- 1/4 cucumber, sliced
- 1/4 red onion, thinly sliced
- 1/4 cup crumbled feta cheese (optional)
- 2 tablespoons lemon juice
- 1 tablespoon olive oil
- 1/2 teaspoon Dijon mustard
- 1/4 teaspoon dried oregano
- Salt and pepper to taste

Directions:

1. Marinate the chicken: In a bowl, combine olive oil, salt, and pepper. Rub the mixture onto the chicken breast and let it marinate for at least 10 minutes.
2. Grill the chicken: Preheat your grill to medium-high heat. Grill the chicken breast for 7-8 minutes per side, or until cooked through. Let the chicken cool slightly and then shred it with two forks.
3. Prepare the salad: In a large bowl, combine mixed greens, cherry tomatoes, cucumber, and red onion.
4. Make the dressing: In a small bowl, whisk together lemon juice, olive oil, Dijon mustard, oregano, salt, and pepper.
5. Assemble the salad: Add the shredded chicken to the salad bowl. Drizzle with the dressing and toss to coat. Top with crumbled feta cheese (optional).

Nutritional Information: Calories: 350, Protein: 35g, Fat: 5g, Carbohydrates: 10g, Fiber: 5g

Tips:
- For added flavor, you can marinate the chicken in your favorite herbs and spices.
- Use a nonstick cooking spray to prevent the chicken from sticking to the grill.
- Serve the salad with a whole-wheat roll or pita bread for extra fiber.
- If you are watching your sodium intake, you can omit the feta cheese or use a low-sodium option.
- You can also substitute other lean protein sources, such as grilled fish or tofu, for the chicken.

Quinoa and Vegetable Stir-Fry

Prep Time: 10 minutes | **Cooking Time**: 20 minutes | **Total Time**: 30 minutes | **Servings**: 2

Ingredients:

- 1 cup quinoa, rinsed
- 2 cups vegetable broth
- 1 tablespoon olive oil
- 1/2 onion, diced
- 2 cloves garlic, minced
- 1 bell pepper, diced
- 1 cup broccoli florets
- 1 cup baby carrots, sliced
- 1/2 cup frozen peas
- 1 tablespoon low-sodium soy sauce
- 1 teaspoon rice vinegar
- 1/2 teaspoon ground ginger
- Salt and pepper to taste

Directions:

1. Cook the quinoa: In a saucepan, combine quinoa and vegetable broth. Bring to a boil, then reduce heat, cover, and simmer for 15 minutes, or until quinoa is fluffy and cooked through. Fluff with a fork and set aside.
2. Sauté the vegetables: Heat olive oil in a large skillet or wok over medium heat. Add onion and cook for 3-4 minutes, until softened. Add garlic and cook for another minute, until fragrant.
3. Add bell pepper, broccoli, and carrots: Stir-fry for 5-7 minutes, until slightly tender.
4. Incorporate remaining ingredients: Add peas, cooked quinoa, soy sauce, rice vinegar, and ginger. Stir-fry for another 2-3 minutes, until peas are heated through and everything is well combined.
5. Season and serve: Season with salt and pepper to taste. Serve immediately and enjoy!

Nutritional Information per Serving: Calories: 350, Fat: 8g, Carbohydrates: 45g, Fiber: 7g, Protein: 15g

Tips:

- For extra protein, add tofu, tempeh, or cooked chicken breast.
- Substitute different vegetables based on your preferences.
- Use low-sodium broth and sauce to keep the sodium content in check.
- Feel free to add a squeeze of fresh lime juice or a sprinkle of chili flakes for extra flavor.
- Store leftovers in an airtight container in the refrigerator for up to 3 days.

Turkey and Avocado Wrap

Cooking Time: None | **Prep Time**: 5 minutes | **Total Time**: 5 minutes | **Serving Size**: 1 wrap

Ingredients:

- 1 whole wheat tortilla (8-inch)
- 3 ounces sliced deli turkey breast
- 1/4 medium avocado, sliced
- 1/2 cup romaine lettuce, shredded
- 1/4 cup cucumber, sliced
- 1 tablespoon Dijon mustard
- Salt and pepper to taste

Directions:

1. Spread the Dijon mustard evenly over the tortilla.

2. Layer the turkey, avocado, lettuce, and cucumber on one half of the tortilla.

3. Season with salt and pepper to taste.

4. Fold the tortilla in half and roll up tightly.

5. Enjoy!

Nutritional Information per serving: Calories: 340, Fat: 12g, Carbs: 18g, Fiber: 4g, Protein: 30g

Tips:

- For extra flavor, toast the tortilla lightly in a dry pan before assembling the wrap.
- Substitute Greek yogurt for the Dijon mustard for a lighter option.
- Add a sprinkle of dried cranberries or chopped nuts for extra crunch.
- Use a low-sodium deli turkey to reduce the sodium content.
- Serve with a side of fruit or salad for a complete meal.

Lentil Soup

Prep Time: 10 minutes | **Cooking Time**: 30 minutes | **Total Time**: 40 minutes | **Serving Size**: 4 servings

Ingredients:

- 1 tablespoon olive oil
- 1 onion, chopped
- 2 carrots, chopped
- 2 celery stalks, chopped
- 2 cloves garlic, minced
- 1 teaspoon ground cumin
- 1/2 teaspoon ground coriander
- 1/4 teaspoon chili powder (optional)
- 4 cups vegetable broth
- 1 cup brown lentils, rinsed
- 1 (14.5oz) can diced tomatoes, undrained
- 1 cup chopped kale or spinach
- Salt and pepper to taste

Directions:

1. Heat olive oil in a large pot over medium heat. Add onion, carrots, and celery and cook until softened, about 5 minutes.

2. Add garlic, cumin, coriander, and chili powder (if using) and cook for another minute, until fragrant.

3. Add vegetable broth, lentils, and diced tomatoes with their juices. Bring to a boil, then reduce heat, cover, and simmer for 20 minutes, or until lentils are tender.

4. Stir in kale or spinach and cook until wilted. Season with salt and pepper to taste.

5. Serve hot and enjoy!

Nutritional Information per Serving: Calories: 250, Fat: 3g, Carbs: 34g, Fiber: 12g, Protein: 18g

Tips:

- For a thicker soup, mash some of the lentils before serving.
- Add a squeeze of lemon juice for extra brightness.
- Garnish with fresh herbs like cilantro or parsley.
- You can also add other vegetables like chopped zucchini or bell peppers.
- To make this soup vegan, use vegan vegetable broth and omit the cheese garnish.

Tuna Salad Lettuce Wraps

Cooking Time: None | **Prep Time**: 10 minutes | **Total Time**: 10 minutes | **Serving Size**: 2 wraps

Ingredients:

- 6 oz canned tuna in water, drained and flaked
- 2 tbsp plain Greek yogurt
- 1 tbsp light mayonnaise
- 1/2 stalk celery, finely chopped
- 1/4 red onion, finely chopped
- 1 tbsp Dijon mustard
- 1 tsp lemon juice
- 1/4 tsp dried dill
- Salt and black pepper to taste
- 4 large romaine lettuce leaves, washed and dried

Directions:

1. In a medium bowl, combine the tuna, Greek yogurt, mayonnaise, celery, red onion, Dijon mustard, lemon juice, and dill. Season with salt and pepper to taste.

2. Divide the tuna salad mixture evenly among the lettuce leaves. Wrap the lettuce leaves around the filling, creating tight wraps.

3. Serve immediately.

Nutritional Information per wrap: Calories: 230, Carbs: 6g, Fat: 7g, Protein: 30g

Tips:

- For extra flavor, add a sprinkle of chopped fresh herbs, such as chives or parsley.
- If you prefer a creamier texture, use more Greek yogurt or mayonnaise.
- If you don't have Dijon mustard, you can use regular mustard or another type of mustard.
- To make the wraps ahead of time, prepare the tuna salad and store it in the refrigerator for up to 3 days. Assemble the wraps just before serving.
- Choose romaine lettuce for sturdier wraps, but butter lettuce or other leafy greens can also be used.
- If you're looking for a vegan option, use crumbled tofu instead of tuna.

Veggie and Hummus Wrap

Cooking Time: None | **Prep Time**: 10 minutes | **Total Time**: 10 minutes | **Serving Size**: 1 wrap

Ingredients:

- 1 whole-wheat tortilla (medium size)
- 1/3 cup hummus (plain or roasted red pepper)
- 1/2 cup mixed greens (spinach, romaine, arugula)
- 1/4 cucumber, thinly sliced
- 1/4 red bell pepper, thinly sliced
- 1/4 tomato, thinly sliced
- 1/4 avocado, thinly sliced (optional)
- Salt and pepper to taste

Directions:

1. Wash and chop all vegetables.

2. Spread hummus evenly on half of the tortilla, leaving a 1-inch border around the edge.

3. Layer the mixed greens, cucumber, red pepper, and tomato on top of the hummus.

4. If using avocado, top with avocado slices.

5. Season with salt and pepper to taste.

6. Carefully fold the bottom edge of the tortilla over the filling, then fold in the sides.

7. Roll the tortilla tightly, starting from the bottom.

8. Cut the wrap in half and enjoy!

Nutritional Information per serving: Calories: 300-350, Fat: 5-10g, Carbohydrates: 30-35g, Fiber: 5-7g, Protein: 10-15g

Tips:

- Use a low-fat or reduced-sodium hummus for further calorie reduction.
- Add a sprinkle of crumbled feta cheese or goat cheese for additional protein and flavor (not included in nutritional information).
- Toast the tortilla lightly for a crispier texture.
- Pack this wrap for lunch or a quick and healthy snack.
- For more variety, add other shredded vegetables like carrots, zucchini, or cabbage.
- Feel free to customize the vegetables based on your preferences.

Salmon and Asparagus

Prep Time: 10 minutes | **Cooking Time**: 15 minutes | **Total Time**: 25 minutes | **Serving Size**: 1 person

Ingredients:

- 4 oz. skinless salmon fillet
- 10-12 asparagus spears, trimmed
- 1 tbsp olive oil
- 1/2 tsp dried thyme
- 1/4 tsp garlic powder
- Salt and pepper to taste
- Lemon wedges (optional, for serving)

Directions:

1. Preheat oven to 400°F (200°C).

2. In a small bowl, combine olive oil, thyme, garlic powder, salt, and pepper. Toss asparagus spears in the mixture to coat evenly.

3. Place asparagus spears on one side of a baking sheet. Lay salmon fillet skin-side down on the other side.

4. Bake for 15 minutes, or until salmon is cooked through and flakes easily with a fork. Asparagus should be tender-crisp.

5. Serve immediately with a lemon wedge for squeezing, if desired.

Nutritional Information per Serving: Calories: 350, Protein: 30g, Fat: 15g, Carbs: 5g

Tips:

- For added flavor, you can marinate the salmon in olive oil, lemon juice, and herbs for 15-30 minutes before baking.
- To ensure even cooking, use a baking sheet lined with parchment paper.
- If you prefer your asparagus softer, bake for an additional 5 minutes.
- This recipe is easily doubled or tripled to feed more people.
- Feel free to add a side of quinoa or brown rice for additional complex carbohydrates.

Chickpea Salad

Prep Time: 10 minutes | **Cooking Time**: 0 minutes | **Total Time**: 10 minutes | **Servings**: 2

Ingredients:

- 1 (15 oz) can chickpeas, drained and rinsed
- 1 cucumber, diced
- 1 tomato, diced
- 1/2 red onion, finely chopped
- 1/4 cup crumbled feta cheese (optional for more protein)
- 1/4 cup Kalamata olives, pitted and halved
- 2 tablespoons olive oil
- 1 tablespoon lemon juice
- 1/2 teaspoon dried oregano
- Salt and pepper to taste

Directions:

1. In a large bowl, combine the chickpeas, cucumber, tomato, red onion, and feta cheese (if using).

2. In a small bowl, whisk together the olive oil, lemon juice, oregano, salt, and pepper.

3. Pour the dressing over the chickpea mixture and toss to coat evenly.

4. Stir in the Kalamata olives.

5. Serve immediately or refrigerate for up to 3 days.

Nutritional Information: Calories: 250 per serving, Protein: 15g per serving, Fiber: 8g per serving, Carbs: 20g per serving, Fat: 8g per serving

Tips:

- If you prefer a softer texture for the chickpeas, mash them slightly with a fork before adding them to the salad.
- For a spicy kick, add a pinch of red pepper flakes to the dressing.
- Feel free to customize this recipe with other vegetables you enjoy, such as bell peppers, celery, or carrots.
- You can use chopped fresh herbs, such as parsley or dill, for added flavor.
- Make sure to choose a light feta cheese or omit it altogether to keep the calorie count lower.
- If you don't have Kalamata olives, you can use any type of black olive.

Greek Yogurt Chicken Salad

Prep Time: 10 minutes | **Cooking Time**: 10 minutes | **Total Time**: 20 minutes | **Serving Size**: 1 person

Ingredients:

- 1 cup cooked, shredded chicken breast (about 4 oz)
- 1/2 cup plain nonfat Greek yogurt
- 1/4 cup diced celery
- 1/4 cup chopped red onion
- 1 tablespoon Dijon mustard
- 1 teaspoon lemon juice
- 1/4 teaspoon dried dill
- Salt and pepper to taste

Directions:

1. Cook the chicken: You can use various methods depending on your preference and time constraints:
   - Poach: Bring a pot of water to a boil, then reduce heat and simmer for 10-12 minutes.
   - Bake: Preheat oven to 400°F (200°C). Bake chicken breasts for 20-25 minutes, or until cooked through.
   - Grill: Grill chicken breasts for 15-20 minutes per side, or until cooked through.
   - Use leftover rotisserie chicken: This is a quick and convenient option.
2. Shred the chicken: Once cooked, shred the chicken breast with two forks or use a hand mixer with paddle attachment.
3. Combine ingredients: In a large bowl, combine shredded chicken, Greek yogurt, celery, red onion, Dijon mustard, lemon juice, dill, salt, and pepper.
4. Mix well: Gently toss all ingredients until well combined. Be careful not to over mix, as the chicken can become mushy.
5. Serve: Enjoy your Greek yogurt chicken salad on its own, with lettuce wraps, whole-wheat crackers, or atop a bed of greens.

Nutritional Information per Serving: Calories: 300, Fat: 6g, Saturated Fat: 2g, Carbohydrates: 5g, Sugar: 2g, Protein: 35g, Fiber: 1g

Tips:

- For additional flavor, you can add a pinch of red pepper flakes or garlic powder.
- If you prefer a smoother consistency, you can blend a small portion of the chicken salad with additional Greek yogurt.
- Store leftover chicken salad in an airtight container in the refrigerator for up to 3 days.

Vegetable and Tofu Stir-Fry

Prep Time: 10 minutes | **Cooking Time**: 15 minutes | **Total Time**: 25 minutes | **Servings**: 2

Ingredients:

- 14 oz extra firm tofu, drained and pressed
- 1 tbsp low-sodium soy sauce
- 1 tsp cornstarch
- 1 tsp sesame oil
- 1 tbsp olive oil
- 1 cup broccoli florets
- 1 cup bell peppers (any color), sliced
- 1 cup snap peas, trimmed
- 1 cup sliced carrots
- 1/2 cup sliced onion
- 2 cloves garlic, minced
- 1/2 inch ginger, grated
- 1/4 cup water or vegetable broth
- 1 tbsp chopped fresh cilantro (optional)

Directions:

1. Marinate the tofu: Cut the tofu into cubes and place it in a shallow dish. Combine soy sauce, cornstarch, and sesame oil, and pour over the tofu. Marinate for at least 15 minutes.
2. Prepare the vegetables: While the tofu marinates, wash and chop all the vegetables according to their size and cooking time (broccoli florets should be slightly larger than snap peas).
3. Cook the tofu: Heat olive oil in a large wok or pan over medium-high heat. Add the tofu cubes and cook, stirring occasionally, until golden brown on all sides, about 5-7 minutes. Remove the tofu from the pan and set aside.
4. Stir-fry the vegetables: Add a little more oil to the pan, if needed. Add the onions and garlic, and cook for 1 minute until fragrant. Add the bell peppers and carrots, and stir-fry for 2-3 minutes until slightly softened.
5. Add remaining vegetables and sauce: Next, add the broccoli florets and snap peas. Stir-fry for another 2-3 minutes until crisp-tender. Pour in the water or vegetable broth and bring to a simmer.
6. Incorporate the tofu: Return the cooked tofu to the pan and toss to coat in the sauce. Cook for another minute to heat through.
7. Finish and serve: Turn off the heat and stir in the fresh cilantro (if using). Serve immediately with brown rice or quinoa for a complete meal.

Nutritional Information per Serving: Calories: 350, Fat: 10g, Carbohydrates: 30g, Fiber: 8g, Protein: 20g

Tips:

- Adjust the vegetables to your liking. You can also add other low-calorie options like baby corn, mushrooms, or zucchini.
- Use low-sodium soy sauce or coconut aminos for a reduced sodium alternative.
- Serve with a whole-wheat wrap or lettuce leaves for a low-carb option.
- For added flavor, garnish with a sprinkle of toasted sesame seeds or chili flakes.

Egg Salad Lettuce Cups

Cooking Time: 10 minutes | **Prep Time**: 10 minutes | **Total Time**: 20 minutes | **Serving Size**: 2 cups

Ingredients:

- 4 large eggs
- 1/4 cup plain nonfat Greek yogurt
- 1 tablespoon mayonnaise (light or low-fat)
- 1/2 teaspoon Dijon mustard
- Pinch of salt
- Ground black pepper to taste
- 2 stalks celery, finely chopped
- 2 green onions, thinly sliced
- 4 large romaine lettuce leaves, washed and dried

Directions:

1. Hard-boil the eggs: Place the eggs in a saucepan and cover with cold water. Bring to a boil, then remove from heat and cover with a lid. Let stand for 10 minutes. Drain and run under cold water until cool enough to handle. Peel and discard the shells.

2. Chop the eggs: Roughly chop the eggs and place them in a medium bowl.

3. Make the dressing: In a small bowl, whisk together the Greek yogurt, mayonnaise, Dijon mustard, salt, and pepper until smooth.

4. Combine the ingredients: Add the chopped celery, green onions, and dressing to the eggs and stir gently to combine. Avoid over mixing, as you want some texture in the egg salad.

5. Assemble the lettuce cups: Wash and dry the romaine lettuce leaves. Divide the egg salad mixture evenly among the lettuce leaves.

6. Serve: Enjoy immediately!

Nutritional Information per serving: Calories: 250, Fat: 10g, Carbohydrates: 4g, Fiber: 2g, Protein: 20g

Tips:

- For a spicier version, add a pinch of cayenne pepper or red pepper flakes to the dressing.
- You can use other crunchy vegetables instead of celery, such as cucumber or red bell pepper.
- If you prefer a creamier egg salad, you can mash the eggs instead of chopping them.
- To make this recipe ahead of time, store the egg salad in an airtight container in the refrigerator for up to 3 days. Assemble the lettuce cups just before serving.

Cauliflower Fried Rice

Prep Time: 10 minutes | **Cooking Time**: 15 minutes | **Total Time**: 25 minutes | **Servings**: 2

Ingredients:

- 1 head cauliflower, chopped into florets
- 1 tbsp olive oil
- 1/2 onion, diced
- 1 clove garlic, minced
- 1 carrot, diced
- 1/2 cup frozen peas
- 2 eggs, beaten
- 2 tbsp low-sodium soy sauce
- 1/2 tsp sesame oil
- 1/4 tsp ground ginger
- Salt and pepper to taste
- Chopped green onions (optional, for garnish)

Directions:

1. Prepare the cauliflower rice: Pulse the cauliflower florets in a food processor until they resemble rice-like grains. Alternatively, grate the cauliflower using the large holes of a box grater.

2. Heat the oil in a large skillet or wok over medium heat. Add the onion and cook until softened, about 3 minutes. Add the garlic and cook for another minute.

3. Add the carrots and peas to the pan and cook for 3-4 minutes, until slightly softened.

4. Push the vegetables to the side of the pan and add the beaten eggs. Scramble the eggs until cooked through, then combine with the vegetables.

5. Stir in the cauliflower rice, soy sauce, sesame oil, and ginger. Cook for 5-7 minutes, until the cauliflower rice is heated through.

6. Season with salt and pepper to taste. Garnish with chopped green onions (optional).

Nutritional Information per Serving: Calories: 250, Carbs: 15g, Fat: 10g, Protein: 10g, Fiber: 4g

Tips:

- For a more flavorful cauliflower rice, toast it in a dry skillet before adding it to the pan.
- Feel free to use other vegetables of your choice, such as broccoli, bell peppers, or zucchini.
- You can use tofu scramble instead of eggs for a vegan option.
- Serve with a side of grilled chicken or shrimp for a complete meal.

Turkey and Bean Chili

Prep Time: 15 minutes | **Cooking Time**: 30 minutes | **Total Time**: 45 minutes | **Servings**: 4

Ingredients:

- 1 tablespoon olive oil
- 1 medium onion, chopped
- 1 green bell pepper, chopped
- 2 cloves garlic, minced
- 1 pound ground turkey breast (93% lean)
- 1 tablespoon chili powder
- 1 teaspoon ground cumin
- 1/2 teaspoon dried oregano
- 1/4 teaspoon black pepper
- 1 (28-ounce) can crushed tomatoes, undrained
- 1 (15-ounce) can black beans, rinsed and drained
- 1 (15-ounce) can kidney beans, rinsed and drained
- 1 cup low-sodium chicken broth
- 1/2 cup chopped fresh cilantro

Directions:

1. Heat olive oil in a large pot or Dutch oven over medium heat. Add onion and bell pepper, and cook for 5 minutes, or until softened. Add garlic and cook for an additional minute.

2. Add ground turkey and break up with a spoon as it cooks. Cook until browned and no longer pink.

3. Stir in chili powder, cumin, oregano, and black pepper. Cook for 1 minute, stirring constantly, to toast the spices.

4. Add crushed tomatoes, black beans, kidney beans, and chicken broth. Bring to a boil, then reduce heat and simmer for 20 minutes, or until chili thickens slightly.

5. Stir in fresh cilantro and serve immediately.

Nutritional Information per serving: Calories: 350, Fat: 8g, Carbs: 40g, Fiber: 12g, Protein: 30g

Tips:

- For a spicier chili, add a pinch of cayenne pepper or a diced jalapeño with the other vegetables.
- You can substitute ground chicken breast for the ground turkey.
- Serve with chopped avocado, low-fat Greek yogurt, or a dollop of salsa for added flavor and nutrients.
- Store leftovers in an airtight container in the refrigerator for up to 3 days.

Caprese Salad

Prep Time: 5 minutes | **Cooking Time**: 0 minutes | **Total Time**: 5 minutes | **Servings**: 1

Ingredients:

- 1 medium tomato, sliced
- 1/2 cup cherry tomatoes, halved
- 4-5 slices fresh mozzarella cheese (about 50g)
- 5-6 fresh basil leaves, torn
- 1 tablespoon extra-virgin olive oil
- Salt and freshly ground black pepper, to taste

Directions:

1. Wash and slice the tomato. If using cherry tomatoes, simply halve them.

2. Slice the mozzarella cheese into thin slices.

3. Arrange the tomato slices and cherry tomatoes on a plate.

4. Top with the mozzarella cheese slices.

5. Scatter the torn basil leaves on top.

6. Drizzle with extra virgin olive oil.

7. Season with salt and freshly ground black pepper to taste.

8. Serve immediately.

Nutritional Information per serving: Calories: 220, Fat: 12g, Carbs: 10g, Fiber: 2g, Protein: 14g, Sodium: 280mg (depending on cheese)

Tips:

- For a lower-sodium option, choose low-sodium mozzarella cheese.
- Want more protein? Add a grilled chicken breast or shrimp on top.
- Drizzle with balsamic vinegar for a tangy twist.
- Use a variety of colored cherry tomatoes for added visual appeal.
- Serve with whole-wheat bread or crackers for a more filling meal.

Veggie and Bean Burrito Bowl

Prep Time: 15 minutes | **Cooking Time**: 20 minutes | **Total Time**: 35 minutes | **Serving Size**: 1 person

Ingredients:

Base:
- 1/2 cup brown rice, cooked
- 1/2 cup mixed greens (spinach, kale, and romaine)

Beans:
- 1/2 cup black beans, rinsed and drained
- 1/4 tsp ground cumin
- 1/4 tsp chili powder
- 1/8 tsp garlic powder
- Pinch of salt and pepper

Veggies:
- 1/2 bell pepper, diced
- 1/2 cup broccoli florets
- 1/4 cup cherry tomatoes
- 1/4 cup red onion, diced

Toppings:
- 1/4 avocado, sliced
- 1 tbsp fresh cilantro, chopped
- 1 lime wedge
- 1 tbsp salsa (optional)
- Hot sauce (optional)

Directions:

1. Cook the rice: Rinse and cook the brown rice according to package instructions. Set aside to cool slightly.
2. Season the beans: Combine black beans, cumin, chili powder, garlic powder, salt, and pepper in a small bowl. Mix well.
3. Roast the vegetables: Preheat oven to 400°F (200°C). Spread bell pepper, broccoli, and red onion on a baking sheet. Roast for 15-20 minutes, or until tender-crisp.
4. Assemble the bowl: Divide cooked rice, mixed greens, seasoned beans, and roasted vegetables between two bowls.
5. Top with avocado, cilantro, and a squeeze of lime juice.
6. Optional: Add salsa and hot sauce for additional flavor and heat.

Nutritional Information per Serving: Calories: 400, Fat: 8g, Saturated Fat: 2g, Carbohydrates: 45g, Fiber: 10g, Sugars: 10g (naturally occurring), Protein: 15g

Tips:

- Use other low-calorie grains like quinoa or barley instead of brown rice.
- Add other lean protein options like grilled chicken breast or tofu for more protein.
- For a spicier version, add chopped jalapeño to the salsa or avocado.
- You can prep the bean mixture, roasted vegetables, and rice in advance for quick and easy assembly.
- Adjust the toppings to your liking and dietary preferences.

Shrimp and Zucchini Noodles

Cooking Time: 15 minutes | **Prep Time**: 10 minutes | **Total Time**: 25 minutes | **Serving Size**: 1

Ingredients:

- 4oz medium shrimp, peeled and deveined
- 1 medium zucchini, spiralized
- 1 tablespoon olive oil
- 2 cloves garlic, minced
- 1/4 teaspoon dried oregano
- 1/4 teaspoon red pepper flakes (optional)
- 1/4 cup dry white wine or chicken broth
- 1/4 cup cherry tomatoes, halved (optional)
- 1 tablespoon lemon juice
- Fresh parsley, chopped, for garnish

Directions:

1. Prep: Wash and spiralize the zucchini. Set aside. Peel and devein the shrimp, removing any tails.
2. Cook Shrimp: Heat olive oil in a large skillet over medium heat. Add shrimp and cook, stirring occasionally, until pink and opaque, about 2-3 minutes. Remove from the pan and set aside.
3. Garlic and Herbs: Add garlic, oregano, and red pepper flakes (if using) to the pan and cook until fragrant, about 30 seconds.
4. Zucchini Noodles: Add zucchini noodles to the pan and cook, stirring frequently, for 2-3 minutes until slightly softened. Do not overcook, as they will become mushy.
5. Deglaze and Flavor: Pour in white wine or broth and scrape up any browned bits from the bottom of the pan. Add cherry tomatoes (if using) and simmer for 1 minute.
6. Return Shrimp: Add shrimp back to the pan with lemon juice. Toss to coat shrimp in the flavorful sauce and heat through, about 1 minute.
7. Garnish and Serve: Plate the zucchini noodles and shrimp mixture. Garnish with fresh parsley and enjoy.

Tips:

- For a richer flavor, add a tablespoon of butter along with the olive oil when cooking the shrimp.
- Serve with a side of steamed broccoli or spinach for additional nutrients.
- If you don't have dry white wine, you can use chicken broth for a similar flavor.
- Adjust the amount of red pepper flakes to your desired level of spiciness.
- Feel free to add other vegetables like chopped bell peppers or mushrooms to the dish for extra variety.

Turkey and Vegetable Lettuce Wraps

Prep Time: 10 minutes | **Cooking Time**: 15 minutes | **Total Time**: 25 minutes | **Servings**: 4

Ingredients:

- 1 pound ground turkey (90% lean or higher)
- 1 onion, chopped
- 1 bell pepper, chopped
- 1 cup broccoli florets
- 1/2 cup carrot, shredded
- 1/4 cup water
- 2 tablespoons soy sauce
- 1 tablespoon rice vinegar
- 1 teaspoon sesame oil
- 1/2 teaspoon ground ginger
- 1/4 teaspoon garlic powder
- 1/4 teaspoon black pepper
- 1 head romaine lettuce, leaves separated and washed

Directions:

1. Prep: Wash and chop all vegetables. In a small bowl, whisk together soy sauce, rice vinegar, sesame oil, ginger, garlic powder, and black pepper. Set aside.

2. Cook turkey: Heat a large skillet over medium heat. Add ground turkey and cook until browned, breaking it up with a spoon. Drain any excess grease.

3. Add vegetables: Add onion, bell pepper, broccoli, and carrot to the skillet with the turkey. Stir-fry for 5 minutes, or until vegetables are softened but still slightly crisp.

4. Sauce and simmer: Pour in the reserved sauce mixture and stir to coat the vegetables and turkey. Bring to a simmer and cook for 2-3 minutes, or until sauce thickens slightly.

5. Assemble: Spoon turkey mixture into romaine lettuce leaves. Serve immediately.

Tips:

- For added flavor, you can brown the ground turkey with a drizzle of olive oil before adding the vegetables.
- To make the wraps even more filling, add cooked quinoa or brown rice to the lettuce leaves before adding the turkey mixture.
- If you prefer a spicier wrap, add a pinch of red pepper flakes to the sauce mixture.
- For a vegetarian option, substitute ground turkey with crumbled tofu.
- Store leftover filling in an airtight container in the refrigerator for up to 3 days.

Stuffed Bell Peppers

Cooking Time: 40 minutes | **Prep Time**: 15 minutes | **Total Time**: 55 minutes | **Serving Size**: 4 peppers

Ingredients:

- 4 medium bell peppers (any color)
- 1 pound lean ground turkey
- 1/2 cup chopped onion
- 1 cup chopped mushrooms
- 1/2 cup diced zucchini
- 1/4 cup chopped fresh parsley
- 1 clove garlic, minced
- 1 tsp chili powder
- 1/2 tsp cumin
- 1/4 tsp smoked paprika
- 1 (14.5 oz) can diced tomatoes, undrained
- 1/2 cup low-fat shredded mozzarella cheese

Directions:

- Preheat oven to 375°F (190°C). Prepare the bell peppers by washing, cutting off the tops, and removing the seeds and membranes. Place the peppers upright in a baking dish.
- Brown the ground turkey in a large skillet over medium heat. Break up the meat with a spoon and cook until browned. Drain any excess fat.
- Add onion, mushrooms, and zucchini to the skillet and cook for 5 minutes, or until softened. Stir in garlic, chili powder, cumin, and paprika, and cook for an additional minute.
- Stir in diced tomatoes and parsley to the skillet. Bring to a simmer and cook for 5 minutes.
- Spoon the filling evenly into the prepared bell peppers. Sprinkle each pepper with shredded cheese.
- Cover the baking dish with foil and bake for 30 minutes. Remove the foil and bake for an additional 10 minutes, or until the peppers are tender and the cheese is melted and bubbly.
- Let cool slightly before serving. Enjoy as a complete meal or with a side salad for added fiber and nutrients.

Nutritional Information: Calories: 280, Fat: 7g, Carbs: 25g, Fiber: 5g, Protein: 24g

Tips:

- For a vegetarian option, substitute cooked lentils or black beans for the ground turkey.
- Use brown rice or quinoa instead of ground meat for a higher-fiber filling.
- Top with a dollop of plain Greek yogurt for additional protein and creaminess.
- Add a sprinkle of red pepper flakes for a bit of heat.
- Store leftover stuffed peppers in an airtight container in the refrigerator for up to 3 days.

Spinach and Feta Omelette

Cooking Time: 10 minutes | **Prep Time**: 5 minutes | **Total Time**: 15 minutes | **Serving Size**: 1 omelette

Ingredients:

- 2 large eggs
- 1 tbsp water
- 1/2 cup baby spinach, washed
- 1/4 cup crumbled feta cheese
- Salt and black pepper to taste

Directions:

1. Beat the eggs: In a bowl, whisk together the eggs and water until well combined. Season with salt and pepper.

2. Cook the spinach: Heat a non-stick pan over medium heat. Add the spinach and cook until wilted, about 1-2 minutes.

3. Pour the egg mixture: Add the egg mixture to the pan and swirl the pan to evenly distribute the spinach.

4. Cook the bottom of the omelette: Let the omelette cook undisturbed for about 2-3 minutes, or until the bottom is set.

5. Add the feta cheese: Sprinkle half of the feta cheese over one half of the omelette.

6. Fold the omelette: Use a spatula to fold the other half of the omelette over the cheese.

7. Cook the other side: Continue cooking for another 1-2 minutes, or until the omelette is cooked through.

8. Serve: Slide the omelette onto a plate and sprinkle with the remaining feta cheese.

Tips:

- Use low-fat feta cheese to reduce the calorie and fat content.

- Add other vegetables to the omelette, such as chopped tomatoes, onions, or bell peppers.

- Serve the omelette with a side of fruit or whole-wheat toast.

- For a vegetarian option, use egg substitutes instead of eggs.

Chicken and Vegetable Skewers

Cooking Time: 25-30 minutes | **Prep Time**: 15 minutes | **Total Time**: 30-45 minutes | **Servings**: 4

Ingredients:

- 1 pound boneless, skinless chicken breasts, cut into bite-sized pieces
- 1 medium zucchini, cut into chunks
- 1 bell pepper, any color, cut into chunks
- 1 small red onion, cut into wedges
- 1 tablespoon olive oil
- 1 tablespoon lemon juice
- 1/2 teaspoon dried oregano
- 1/4 teaspoon garlic powder
- 1/4 teaspoon black pepper
- Salt to taste
- 4 wooden skewers, soaked in water for at least 30 minutes

Directions:

1. In a large bowl, combine olive oil, lemon juice, oregano, garlic powder, pepper, and salt. Add chicken pieces and toss to coat evenly. Cover and refrigerate for at least 30 minutes, or up to overnight.
2. Preheat grill to medium-high heat or oven to 400°F (200°C).
3. Thread chicken and vegetables onto soaked skewers, alternating between them.
4. For grilling: Grill skewers for 15-20 minutes, flipping every few minutes, until chicken is cooked through and vegetables are tender.
5. For baking: Arrange skewers on a baking sheet lined with parchment paper. Bake for 25-30 minutes, flipping halfway through, until chicken is cooked through and vegetables are tender.
6. Serve immediately, with a side of brown rice or quinoa and a simple salad for a complete meal.

Nutritional Information: Calories: 250, Fat: 5g, Protein: 35g, Carbohydrates: 10g, Fiber: 3g

Tips:

- You can marinate the chicken in your favorite low-fat marinade instead of the one provided. Just be sure to choose a marinade that is low in sugar and added fats.
- For additional flavor, try adding diced fresh herbs like rosemary or thyme to the marinade.
- If you don't have wooden skewers, you can use metal skewers. Just be sure to soak them in water for at least 30 minutes to prevent them from burning.
- To make the skewers even more filling, you can add cooked shrimp or tofu to them.
- Feel free to experiment with different types of vegetables, such as mushrooms, asparagus, or cherry tomatoes.

Grilled Lemon Herb Chicken

Cooking Time: 20-25 minutes | **Prep Time**: 10 minutes | **Total Time**: 30-35 minutes | **Serving Size**: 2 servings

Ingredients:

- 2 boneless, skinless chicken breasts (about 6 oz each)
- 2 tablespoons olive oil
- 2 tablespoons lemon juice
- 1 tablespoon fresh thyme leaves, chopped
- 1 tablespoon fresh rosemary leaves, chopped
- 1/2 teaspoon dried oregano
- 1/4 teaspoon garlic powder
- 1/4 teaspoon salt
- 1/4 teaspoon black pepper

Directions:

1. Prepare the marinade: In a bowl, whisk together olive oil, lemon juice, thyme, rosemary, oregano, garlic powder, salt, and pepper.
2. Marinate the chicken: Place chicken breasts in a shallow dish and pour the marinade over them. Cover and refrigerate for at least 30 minutes, or up to 4 hours.
3. Preheat the grill: Preheat your grill to medium-high heat. If using a charcoal grill, ensure the coals are mostly white with some red ash.
4. Grill the chicken: Remove chicken from the marinade and discard the marinade. Place chicken breasts on the preheated grill. Grill for 5-7 minutes per side, or until cooked through and reaching an internal temperature of 165°F.
5. Rest and serve: Transfer the chicken to a plate and let it rest for 5 minutes before slicing and serving.

Nutritional Information: Calories: 250, Protein: 35g, Fat: 5g, Carbohydrates: 2g

Tips:

- For extra flavor, sprinkle the chicken with additional fresh herbs after grilling.
- Serve the chicken with a side of grilled vegetables or a simple salad for a complete meal.
- If you don't have fresh herbs, you can substitute 1 teaspoon each of dried thyme, rosemary, and oregano.
- To make the chicken breasts cook more evenly, pound them to an even thickness before grilling.

Baked Salmon with Dill Sauce

Cooking Time: 20 minutes | **Pre Time** p: 5 minutes | **Total Time**: 25 minutes | **Serving Size**: 1

Ingredients:

- 4 oz skinless salmon fillet
- 1/2 tablespoon olive oil
- 1/4 teaspoon salt
- 1/4 teaspoon black pepper
- 1/4 cup plain Greek yogurt
- 1 tablespoon chopped fresh dill
- 1 tablespoon lemon juice
- 1/2 clove garlic, minced

Directions:

1. Preheat oven to 400°F (200°C). Line a baking sheet with parchment paper.

2. Pat the salmon dry with paper towels. Season with salt and pepper.

3. Place the salmon on the prepared baking sheet. Drizzle with olive oil.

4. Bake for 15-20 minutes, or until the salmon is cooked through and flakes easily with a fork.

5. While the salmon is baking, prepare the dill sauce. In a small bowl, combine Greek yogurt, dill, lemon juice, and garlic. Mix well.

6. Once the salmon is cooked, spoon the dill sauce over the top.

Nutritional Information: Calories: 330, Fat: 13g, Carbs: 3g, Protein: 40g

Tips:

- For a richer sauce, you can use full-fat Greek yogurt instead of plain.

- To add some spice, you can also add a pinch of cayenne pepper to the sauce.

- Serve with roasted vegetables or a side salad for a complete meal.

Stir-Fried Tofu and Vegetables

Prep Time: 10 minutes | **Cooking Time**: 15 minutes | **Total Time**: 25 minutes | **Serving Size**: 2

Ingredients:

- 14 oz firm tofu, drained and cubed
- 1 tbsp low-sodium soy sauce
- 1 tsp sesame oil
- 1/2 tsp ground ginger
- 1/4 tsp garlic powder
- 1 tbsp vegetable oil
- 1 onion, sliced
- 2 cloves garlic, minced
- 2 cups assorted vegetables (e.g., broccoli florets, bell peppers, snap peas, carrots)
- 1/4 cup frozen peas
- 1/4 cup chopped fresh cilantro

Directions:

1. Marinate the tofu: In a bowl, combine the soy sauce, sesame oil, ginger, and garlic powder. Add the tofu cubes and toss to coat. Marinate for at least 10 minutes, while prepping the vegetables.
2. Heat the oil: In a large pan or wok, heat the vegetable oil over medium-high heat.
3. Stir-fry the onion and garlic: Add the onion to the pan and cook until softened, about 3 minutes. Add the garlic and cook for another minute, until fragrant.
4. Add the vegetables: Add the assorted vegetables and stir-fry for 5-7 minutes, or until slightly tender-crisp.
5. Add the tofu and peas: Add the marinated tofu and frozen peas to the pan. Stir-fry for another 2-3 minutes, until the tofu is heated through and the peas are thawed.
6. Finish and serve: Stir in the cilantro and season with salt and pepper to taste. Serve immediately with brown rice or quinoa for a complete meal.

Nutritional Information: Calories: 350, Fat: 10g, Carbohydrates: 25g, Fiber: 8g, Protein: 20g

Tips:

- Use a non-stick pan to prevent sticking and reduce the need for additional oil.
- Customize the vegetables with your favorites! Other low-calorie options include bok choy, mushrooms, zucchini, and cabbage.
- If you prefer a thicker sauce, you can add a cornstarch slurry (1 tbsp cornstarch mixed with 2 tbsp water) to the pan after stirring in the tofu and peas. Cook for an additional minute, until the sauce thickens.
- This recipe is easily doubled or tripled to feed more people.
- For added flavor, you can use low-sodium broth instead of water for the cornstarch slurry.

Zucchini Noodles with Turkey Meatballs

Prep Time: 15 minutes | **Cooking Time**: 25 minutes | **Total Time**: 40 minutes | **Servings**: 2

Ingredients:
Meatballs:

- 1 pound lean ground turkey (93% lean or higher)
- 1/4 cup rolled oats
- 1/4 cup grated Parmesan cheese
- 1 egg, beaten
- 1/2 teaspoon dried oregano
- 1/4 teaspoon garlic powder
- 1/4 teaspoon onion powder
- Salt and pepper to taste

Zucchini Noodles:

- 2 medium zucchinis, spiralized
- 1 tablespoon olive oil
- 1/4 teaspoon dried basil
- Pinch of crushed red pepper flakes (optional)
- Salt and pepper to taste

Sauce (optional):

- 1 cup marinara sauce (sugar-free preferred)

Directions:

1. Make the meatballs: In a large bowl, combine ground turkey, rolled oats, Parmesan cheese, egg, oregano, garlic powder, onion powder, salt, and pepper. Mix well with your hands until everything is evenly incorporated.
2. Form the meatballs: Roll the mixture into 1-inch balls. Place them on a baking sheet lined with parchment paper.
3. Bake the meatballs: Preheat oven to 400°F (200°C). Bake the meatballs for 20-25 minutes, or until cooked through and browned.
4. Prepare the zucchini noodles: Using a spiralizer or mandoline, spiralize the zucchinis into thin noodles. If you don't have a spiralizer, you can julienne the zucchinis with a knife.
5. Cook the zucchini noodles: Heat olive oil in a large skillet over medium heat. Add the zucchini noodles and cook for 2-3 minutes, or until just softened. Season with basil, red pepper flakes (optional), salt, and pepper.
6. Assemble and serve: Divide the zucchini noodles between two plates. Top with the baked turkey meatballs and drizzle with marinara sauce if using.

Nutritional Information: Calories: 350, Fat: 10g, Carbs: 15g, Net Carbs: 5g, , Protein: 30g

Tips:

- For even lighter meatballs, substitute ground turkey breast for ground turkey thigh.
- You can add chopped fresh herbs like parsley or cilantro to the zucchini noodles for extra flavor.
- Use a low-sodium marinara sauce if desired.
- If you don't have rolled oats, you can use breadcrumbs instead. Just make sure to adjust the carb count accordingly.
- Leftovers can be stored in an airtight container in the refrigerator for up to 3 days.

Vegetarian Chili

Cooking Time: 30 minutes | **Prep Time**: 10 minutes | **Total Time**: 40 minutes | **Servings**: 4

Ingredients:

- 1 tablespoon olive oil
- 1 medium onion, chopped
- 1 green bell pepper, chopped
- 2 cloves garlic, minced
- 1 teaspoon chili powder
- 1/2 teaspoon cumin
- 1/4 teaspoon smoked paprika
- 1 (28-ounce) can diced tomatoes, undrained
- 1 (15-ounce) can black beans, rinsed and drained
- 1 (15-ounce) can kidney beans, rinsed and drained
- 1 cup vegetable broth
- 1/2 cup frozen corn
- 1/4 cup chopped fresh cilantro (optional)

Directions:

1. Heat olive oil in a large pot over medium heat. Add onion and bell pepper, cook until softened, about 5 minutes.

2. Stir in garlic, chili powder, cumin, and paprika. Cook for another minute until fragrant.

3. Add diced tomatoes, black beans, kidney beans, and vegetable broth. Bring to a boil, then reduce heat and simmer for 20 minutes.

4. Stir in frozen corn and cook for an additional 5 minutes, or until heated through.

5. Season with salt and pepper to taste.

6. Serve hot with your desired toppings, such as chopped avocado, fresh lime wedges, and chopped red onion.

Nutritional Information: Calories: 320, Fat: 7g, Protein: 18g, Fiber: 12g, Carbs: 40g

Tips:

- For a thicker chili, mash some of the beans against the side of the pot with a fork.
- Add a variety of spices to your liking, such as cayenne pepper for heat, oregano for depth, or smoked paprika for a richer flavor.
- Use low-sodium broth and canned beans for a more heart-friendly option.
- Store leftover chili in an airtight container in the refrigerator for up to 3 days.

Grilled Shrimp Skewers with Quinoa Salad

Prep Time: 15 minutes | **Cooking Time**: 15 minutes | **Total Time**: 30 minutes | **Servings**: 2

Ingredients:

For the Shrimp Skewers:
- 1 pound raw shrimp, peeled and deveined
- 1 tablespoon olive oil
- 1/2 teaspoon dried oregano
- 1/4 teaspoon smoked paprika
- 1/4 teaspoon garlic powder
- 1/4 teaspoon black pepper
- 1/8 teaspoon ground cumin
- 1 medium zucchini, cut into 1-inch chunks
- 1 red bell pepper, cut into 1-inch chunks
- 1 yellow bell pepper, cut into 1-inch chunks
- 8 wooden skewers (soaked in water for 30 minutes if using wooden)

For the Quinoa Salad:
- 1 cup dry quinoa, rinsed
- 1 1/2 cups vegetable broth
- 1/4 cup chopped fresh parsley
- 1/4 cup chopped fresh cilantro
- 1/4 cup diced red onion
- 1 tablespoon lemon juice
- 1 tablespoon olive oil
- Salt and pepper to taste

Directions:

1. Marinate the shrimp: In a bowl, combine olive oil, oregano, paprika, garlic powder, black pepper, and cumin. Add shrimp and toss to coat. Marinate for 15 minutes at room temperature.
2. Cook the quinoa: In a saucepan, combine quinoa and vegetable broth. Bring to a boil, then reduce heat, cover, and simmer for 15 minutes or until quinoa is fluffy and liquid is absorbed. Fluff with a fork and set aside to cool.
3. Prepare the salad: While quinoa cools, combine parsley, cilantro, red onion, lemon juice, olive oil, salt, and pepper in a bowl. Add cooled quinoa and toss to combine.
4. Assemble the skewers: Thread shrimp and bell pepper chunks onto the soaked skewers, alternating colors and leaving space between each piece.
5. Grill the skewers: Preheat your grill to medium-high heat. Grill skewers for 3-4 minutes per side, or until shrimp are opaque and cooked through.
6. Serve: Divide quinoa salad between two plates and top with grilled shrimp skewers. Enjoy

Nutritional Information: Calories: 350, Fat: 8g, Carbohydrates: 35g, Fiber: 5g, Protein: 25g

Tips:

- For an extra smoky flavor, add a pinch of smoked paprika to the quinoa salad.
- Feel free to substitute any vegetables you prefer with the bell peppers. Broccoli, asparagus, or cherry tomatoes would be delicious alternatives.
- To make the dish vegan, skip the shrimp and add chickpeas or tofu cubes to the skewers.
- Serve with a side of steamed green beans or a mixed green salad for added fiber and nutrients.

Stuffed Bell Peppers

Prep Time: 20 minutes | **Cooking Time**: 40 minutes | **Total Time**: 60 minutes | **Servings**: 4

Ingredients:

- 4 medium bell peppers (any color)
- 1 pound ground turkey breast
- 1/2 cup diced onion
- 1 clove garlic, minced
- 1 cup brown rice, cooked
- 1 (15 oz) can diced tomatoes, undrained
- 1/2 cup chopped fresh spinach
- 1/4 cup crumbled feta cheese
- 1 teaspoon dried oregano
- 1/2 teaspoon ground cumin
- Salt and pepper to taste

Directions:

1. Preheat oven to 375°F (190°C). Line a baking dish with parchment paper.
2. Prepare the peppers: Wash and halve the bell peppers lengthwise. Remove the seeds and membranes.
3. Cook the ground turkey: In a large skillet over medium heat, brown the ground turkey with the onion and garlic until cooked through. Drain any excess fat.
4. Combine the filling: In a large bowl, combine the cooked ground turkey, brown rice, diced tomatoes, spinach, feta cheese, oregano, cumin, salt, and pepper. Mix well.
5. Stuff the peppers: Divide the filling evenly between the bell pepper halves. Arrange the peppers in the prepared baking dish.
6. Bake: Bake for 40 minutes, or until the peppers are tender and the filling is cooked through.
7. Serve: Enjoy hot with a side salad or steamed vegetables.

Nutritional Information: Calories: 350, Fat: 8g, Carbs: 40g, Fiber: 6g, Protein: 25g

Tips:

- For a vegetarian option, substitute ground tofu or lentils for the ground turkey.
- You can adjust the spices to your preference. Try adding chili powder, smoked paprika, or Italian seasoning.
- For a heartier meal, serve with a whole-wheat roll or pita bread.
- Leftovers can be stored in an airtight container in the refrigerator for up to 3 days.

Cooking Time: 30 minutes | **Prep Time**: 10 minutes | **Total Time**: 40 minutes| **Serving Size**: 1 chicken breast

Ingredients:

- 1 boneless, skinless chicken breast (4-6 oz)
- 1 tablespoon olive oil
- 1 small onion, finely chopped
- 8 oz mushrooms, sliced
- 2 cloves garlic, minced
- 1/2 teaspoon dried thyme
- 1/4 teaspoon black pepper
- 1 cup fresh baby spinach
- 2 tablespoons crumbled feta cheese
- 1 tablespoon chopped fresh parsley

Directions:

1. Preheat oven to 400°F (200°C).
2. Using a sharp knife, carefully make a pocket in the thickest part of the chicken breast. Be careful not to cut all the way through. Season the chicken with salt and pepper.
3. Heat olive oil in a large skillet over medium heat. Add onion and cook until softened, about 5 minutes. Add mushrooms and cook until golden brown, about 5 minutes more. Stir in garlic, thyme, and pepper.
4. Remove from heat and stir in spinach until wilted. Let cool slightly, then stir in feta cheese.
5. Stuff the chicken breast with the mushroom and spinach mixture. Use toothpicks to secure the opening, if needed.
6. Place the chicken breast in a baking dish and bake for 20-25 minutes, or until cooked through and internal temperature reaches 165°F (74°C).
7. Garnish with fresh parsley and serve immediately.

Nutritional Information: Calories: 350, Protein: 35g, Fat: 8g, Carbs: 10g, Fiber: 3g, Sodium: 250mg

Tips:

- For a lighter option, use non-fat feta cheese.
- You can add a squeeze of lemon juice before serving for extra flavor.
- Serve with a side of roasted vegetables or brown rice for a complete meal.
- Feel free to experiment with different herbs and spices in the stuffing.
- To reduce sodium, omit the feta cheese or use a low-sodium version.

Cauliflower Fried Rice

Prep Time: 10 minutes | **Cooking Time**: 15 minutes | **Total Time**: 25 minutes | **Serving Size**: 2

Ingredients:

- 1 head cauliflower, chopped and riced (about 4 cups)
- 1 tbsp olive oil
- 1 egg, beaten
- 1/2 onion, chopped
- 1 clove garlic, minced
- 1 carrot, diced
- 1/2 cup frozen peas
- 1/4 cup chopped green bell pepper
- 2 tbsp low-sodium soy sauce
- 1 tbsp rice vinegar
- 1/2 tsp sesame oil
- 1/4 tsp ground ginger
- Salt and pepper to taste

Directions:

1. Prep your cauliflower: Wash and chop the cauliflower head into florets. Pulse the florets in a food processor or blender until they resemble rice-like grains. Don't over process, as the cauliflower should still have some texture.
2. Heat the oil: In a large skillet or wok, heat olive oil over medium heat.
3. Scramble the egg: Add the beaten egg to the pan and cook, stirring constantly, until scrambled and set. Remove from the pan and set aside.
4. Sauté the aromatics: Add the onion and garlic to the pan and cook for 2-3 minutes, until softened.
5. Add the vegetables: Add the carrot, peas, and bell pepper to the pan and cook for another 3-4 minutes, until slightly softened.
6. Cook the cauliflower rice: Add the riced cauliflower to the pan and cook for 5-7 minutes, stirring frequently, until tender-crisp.
7. Combine and season: Add the scrambled egg, soy sauce, rice vinegar, sesame oil, and ginger to the pan. Toss to combine and cook for another 1-2 minutes, until heated through.
8. Season and serve: Season the rice with salt and pepper to taste. Serve immediately while hot.

Nutritional Information: Calories: 220, Carbs: 15g, Net Carbs: 8g, Fat: 8g, Protein: 10g, Fiber: 4g

Tips:

- For added protein, you can add cooked shrimp, chicken, or tofu to the rice.
- If you don't have a food processor, you can finely grate the cauliflower using a box grater.
- To make the rice even lower in carbs, use cauliflower florets instead of riced cauliflower. Just chop them into small, bite-sized pieces.
- You can use coconut aminos instead of soy sauce for a soy-free option.
- Store leftover rice in an airtight container in the refrigerator for up to 3 days.

Baked Cod with Tomato and Olive Relish

Cooking Time: 20-25 minutes | **Prep Time**: 10 minutes | **Total Time**: 30-35 minutes | **Serving Size**: 1 person

Ingredients:

- 1 (6-oz) cod fillet, skinless and boneless
- 1 medium tomato, chopped
- 1/2 cup pitted Kalamata olives, halved
- 1/4 red onion, finely chopped
- 1 clove garlic, minced
- 1 tablespoon olive oil
- 1 tablespoon lemon juice
- 1/2 teaspoon dried oregano
- 1/4 teaspoon salt
- 1/4 teaspoon black pepper
- Fresh parsley, chopped (for garnish)

Directions:

1. Preheat oven to 400°F (200°C). Lightly grease a baking dish with cooking spray.
2. Pat the cod fillet dry with paper towels and season with salt and pepper. Place the cod in the prepared baking dish.
3. In a bowl, combine chopped tomato, olives, red onion, garlic, olive oil, lemon juice, oregano, salt, and pepper. Mix well.
4. Spread the tomato mixture over the cod fillet.
5. Bake for 20-25 minutes, or until the cod is cooked through and flakes easily with a fork.
6. Garnish with fresh parsley, if desired.

Nutritional Information: Calories: 350, Fat: 8g, Saturated Fat: 2g, Carbohydrates: 15g, Fiber: 2g, Sugar: 5g, Protein: 35g

Tips:

- For an extra boost of flavor, marinate the cod in the lemon juice and herbs for 15 minutes before baking.
- Serve with roasted vegetables, such as broccoli, asparagus, or zucchini, for a complete and balanced meal.
- You can substitute other types of white fish, such as tilapia or halibut, for the cod.
- If you are watching your sodium intake, be sure to choose low-sodium olives.
- This recipe is naturally gluten-free.

Turkey and Vegetable Lettuce Wraps

Cooking Time: 15 minutes | **Prep Time**: 10 minutes | **Total Time**: 25 minutes | **Serving Size**: 2 wraps

Ingredients:

- 1 pound ground turkey breast
- 1/2 cup chopped onion
- 1 clove garlic, minced
- 1 cup chopped bell pepper (any color)
- 1 cup chopped mushrooms
- 1/2 cup chopped carrots
- 1/4 cup low-sodium soy sauce
- 1 tablespoon rice vinegar
- 1 teaspoon sesame oil
- 1/2 teaspoon ground ginger
- 1/4 teaspoon red pepper flakes (optional)
- 4 large romaine lettuce leaves, washed and dried

Directions:

1. In a large skillet, heat oil over medium heat. Add the ground turkey and cook until browned, breaking it up with a spoon. Drain any excess grease.
2. Add the onion, garlic, bell pepper, mushrooms, and carrots to the skillet. Cook for 5-7 minutes, or until the vegetables are softened.
3. In a small bowl, whisk together the soy sauce, rice vinegar, sesame oil, and ginger. Pour the sauce into the skillet and stir to coat the vegetables and turkey. Bring to a simmer and cook for 2-3 minutes, or until the sauce is thickened.
4. Remove the skillet from the heat and let the mixture cool slightly.
5. Divide the filling between the romaine lettuce leaves. Serve immediately.

Nutritional Information: Calories: 300, Fat: 7g, Carbs: 15g, Fiber: 4g, Protein: 25g

Tips:

- For a spicier wrap, add a pinch of red pepper flakes to the sauce.
- You can use any type of ground turkey you like, such as lean ground turkey or ground turkey breast.
- If you don't have romaine lettuce, you can use another type of lettuce, such as butter lettuce or iceberg lettuce.
- Serve these lettuce wraps with your favorite toppings, such as chopped avocado, salsa, or low-fat yogurt.
- Be mindful of portion sizes, as two wraps are considered one serving.

Spaghetti Squash with Turkey Bolognese

Prep Time: 15 minutes | **Cooking Time**: 50 minutes | **Total Time**: 65 minutes | **Servings**: 2

Ingredients:

- 1 medium spaghetti squash (about 3-4 pounds)
- 1 tablespoon olive oil
- 1/2 pound ground turkey breast
- 1/2 onion, finely chopped
- 1 carrot, finely chopped
- 2 cloves garlic, minced
- 1 (28-ounce) can crushed tomatoes
- 1 tablespoon tomato paste
- 1/2 teaspoon dried oregano
- 1/4 teaspoon dried basil
- 1/4 teaspoon red pepper flakes (optional)
- Salt and black pepper to taste
- Fresh basil leaves, for garnish (optional)

Directions:

1. Preheat oven to 400°F (200°C).
2. Prepare the spaghetti squash: Cut the squash in half lengthwise. Scoop out the seeds and discard. Brush the flesh with olive oil and season with salt and pepper. Place the squash halves cut-side down on a baking sheet lined with parchment paper.
3. Bake for 40-50 minutes, or until tender enough to shred with a fork. Let cool slightly.
4. While the squash cooks, prepare the Bolognese: Heat olive oil in a large skillet over medium heat. Add the ground turkey and cook, breaking it up with a spoon, until browned.
5. Add the onion, carrot, and garlic to the skillet and cook for 3-4 minutes, or until softened.
6. Stir in the crushed tomatoes, tomato paste, oregano, basil, and red pepper flakes (if using). Season with salt and pepper to taste. Bring to a simmer and cook for 20 minutes, stirring occasionally.
7. Once the squash is cool enough to handle, use a fork to shred the flesh into spaghetti-like strands.
8. Divide the spaghetti squash between two plates and top with the Bolognese sauce.** Garnish with fresh basil leaves, if desired.

Nutritional Information per Serving: Calories: 380, Fat: 7g, Carbohydrates: 25g (Net Carbs: 7g), Protein: 34g

Tips:
- For an extra boost of flavor, add a handful of chopped mushrooms to the Bolognese sauce.
- To make the dish even lighter, use lean ground turkey (93% lean).
- Leftovers can be stored in an airtight container in the refrigerator for up to 3 days.
- This recipe is easily customizable. Feel free to experiment with different herbs and spices to create your own flavor profile.

Cabbage and Beef Stir-Fry

Prep Time: 15 minutes | **Cooking Time**: 15 minutes | **Total Time**: 30 minutes | **Servings**: 2

Ingredients:

- 1 tablespoon canola oil
- 1/2 pound lean ground beef (90% lean or higher)
- 1/2 small onion, diced
- 2 cloves garlic, minced
- 1 inch ginger, grated
- 4 cups shredded green cabbage
- 1 cup shredded carrots
- 1/4 cup low-sodium soy sauce
- 1 tablespoon rice vinegar
- 1/2 teaspoon sesame oil
- 1/4 teaspoon black pepper
- 1/4 cup chopped green onions (optional, for garnish)

Directions

1. Prepare the vegetables: Shred the cabbage and carrots and set aside. Dice the onion, mince the garlic and ginger, and chop the green onions (if using).
2. Cook the beef: Heat the canola oil in a large skillet or wok over medium-high heat. Add the ground beef and cook until browned, breaking it up with a spoon. Drain any excess fat.
3. Add aromatics: Add the onion, garlic, and ginger to the pan and cook for 30 seconds, stirring frequently.
4. Stir-fry the vegetables: Add the shredded cabbage and carrots to the pan and stir-fry for 3-5 minutes, until slightly softened.
5. Make the sauce: In a small bowl, whisk together the soy sauce, rice vinegar, sesame oil, and black pepper.
6. Finish the stir-fry: Pour the sauce over the vegetables and beef and stir-fry for another minute, until heated through.
7. Serve: Divide the stir-fry between two plates and garnish with chopped green onions (optional).

Nutritional Information per Serving: Calories: 350, Fat: 7g, Carbs: 12g, Protein: 30g, Fiber: 4g, Sodium: 300mg (depending on soy sauce)

Tips:

- Use lean ground beef to reduce the fat content.
- Adjust the amount of soy sauce to your taste preference.
- Add other low-calorie vegetables like broccoli, mushrooms, or bell peppers.
- Serve with brown rice or quinoa for a complete meal.
- For a spicy kick, add a pinch of red pepper flakes to the sauce.
- If you don't have rice vinegar, you can substitute with another type of vinegar, like white vinegar or apple cider vinegar.

Blackened Mahi-Mahi with Mango Salsa

Prep Time: 15 minutes | **Cooking Time**: 8 minutes | **Total Time**: 23 minutes | **Serving Size**: 1

Ingredients:

For the Blackened Mahi-Mahi:
- 1 (6-oz) mahi-mahi fillet
- 1 tablespoon olive oil
- 1/2 teaspoon paprika
- 1/2 teaspoon chili powder
- 1/4 teaspoon garlic powder
- 1/4 teaspoon onion powder
- 1/4 teaspoon black pepper
- 1/8 teaspoon cayenne pepper (adjust to your spice preference)

For the Mango Salsa:
- 1/2 mango, diced
- 1/4 red onion, diced
- 1/4 red bell pepper, diced
- 1 tablespoon fresh cilantro, chopped
- 1 tablespoon lime juice
- 1/4 teaspoon salt

Directions:

1. Prepare the blackening seasoning: In a small bowl, combine paprika, chili powder, garlic powder, onion powder, black pepper, and cayenne pepper.
2. Season the mahi-mahi: Pat the fish dry with paper towels. Drizzle with olive oil and rub the blackening seasoning evenly on both sides.
3. Cook the fish: Heat a large skillet over medium-high heat. Add the remaining olive oil and let it shimmer. Carefully place the seasoned fish in the pan and cook for 4 minutes per side, or until opaque and cooked through.
4. Make the mango salsa: While the fish cooks, combine the diced mango, red onion, bell pepper, cilantro, lime juice, and salt in a bowl. Mix well and set aside.
5. Plate and serve: Place the cooked mahi-mahi on a plate and top with the mango salsa. Enjoy!

Nutritional Information: Calories: 320, Fat: 7g, Carbohydrates: 15g, Fiber: 3g, Protein: 38g, Sodium: 230mg (depending on salt used)

Tips:

- You can substitute cod or halibut for the mahi-mahi.
- To reduce sodium, use low-sodium spices or omit the cayenne pepper.
- Serve the fish over a bed of quinoa or brown rice for added fiber and complex carbohydrates.
- For a more robust flavor, marinate the fish in the blackening seasoning for 30 minutes before cooking.
- Adjust the amount of cayenne pepper to your desired level of spiciness.

Lemon Garlic Shrimp Pasta

Cooking Time: 15 minutes | **Prep Time**: 5 minutes | **Total Time**: 20 minutes | **Serving Size**: 1

Ingredients:

- 4 oz whole wheat pasta (such as penne, linguine, or spaghetti)
- 5 oz raw, peeled, and deveined shrimp
- 1 tbsp olive oil
- 2 cloves garlic, minced
- 1/4 cup dry white wine (optional, can substitute with water)
- 1/2 lemon, juiced
- 1/4 cup fresh parsley, chopped
- Salt and pepper to taste

Directions:

1. Cook the pasta: Bring a large pot of salted water to a boil. Add the pasta and cook according to package directions until al dente. Reserve 1/4 cup of the pasta water before draining.
2. Prepare the shrimp: While the pasta is cooking, pat the shrimp dry with paper towels. Season with salt and pepper.
3. Cook the shrimp: Heat the olive oil in a large skillet over medium heat. Add the garlic and cook for 30 seconds until fragrant. Add the shrimp and cook for 2-3 minutes per side, or until pink and cooked through.
4. Make the sauce: Add the white wine (if using) to the pan and deglaze, scraping up any browned bits from the bottom. Let the wine simmer for 1 minute until slightly reduced. Add the lemon juice, reserved pasta water, and parsley. Season with salt and pepper to taste.
5. Combine everything: Add the cooked pasta to the pan with the shrimp and sauce. Toss to coat everything evenly.
6. Serve immediately: Garnish with additional fresh parsley, if desired, and enjoy!

Nutritional Information per serving: Calories: 450, Fat: 15g, Carbohydrates: 40g, Fiber: 5g, Protein: 30g

Tips:

- For a lighter option, use only half the amount of olive oil.
- You can substitute the white wine with chicken broth or vegetable broth for a non-alcoholic version.
- Add a pinch of red pepper flakes for a bit of heat.
- Serve with a side of steamed vegetables for a more balanced meal.

Vegetable and Tofu Curry

Prep Time: 15 minutes | **Cooking Time**: 25 minutes | **Total Time**: 40 minutes | **Serving Size**: 2 servings

Ingredients:

- 1 tablespoon olive oil
- 1 medium onion, diced
- 2 cloves garlic, minced
- 1 tablespoon grated ginger
- 1 teaspoon ground turmeric
- 1 teaspoon ground cumin
- 1/2 teaspoon ground coriander
- 1/4 teaspoon chili powder (optional, for a bit of heat)
- 1 (13.5-ounce) can unsweetened light coconut milk
- 1 cup vegetable broth
- 1 medium bell pepper, diced
- 1 cup broccoli florets
- 1 cup chopped carrots
- 1 package firm tofu, drained and cubed
- 1/2 cup frozen peas
- 1/4 cup chopped fresh cilantro
- Salt and black pepper to taste

Directions:

1. Heat the oil in a large pot or Dutch oven over medium heat. Add the onion and cook until softened, about 5 minutes.
2. Add the garlic, ginger, turmeric, cumin, coriander, and chili powder (if using). Cook for 1 minute, stirring constantly, until fragrant.
3. Pour in the coconut milk and vegetable broth. Bring to a simmer.
4. Add the bell pepper, broccoli, carrots, and tofu. Simmer for 15 minutes, or until the vegetables are tender and the tofu is heated through.
5. Stir in the frozen peas and cook for 2 minutes more.
6. Remove from heat and stir in the cilantro. Season with salt and black pepper to taste.
7. Serve immediately with brown rice or quinoa for a complete meal.

Nutritional Information per Serving: Calories: 350, Fat: 10g, Carbohydrates: 30g, Fiber: 5g, Protein: 20g

Tips:
- To make this even more weight-loss friendly, use low-fat coconut milk and skip the added oil.
- You can add other vegetables to this curry, such as zucchini, eggplant, or spinach.
- For a spicier curry, add a chopped jalapeno pepper or red pepper flakes.
- Feel free to adjust the spices to your liking.

Baked Chicken Parmesan

Cooking Time: 25 minutes | **Prep Time**: 10 minutes | **Total Time**: 35 minutes | **Serving Size**: 1 serving

Ingredients:

- 1 boneless, skinless chicken breast (4-6 oz)
- 1/2 cup whole-wheat breadcrumbs
- 1/4 cup grated Parmesan cheese
- 1 egg, beaten
- 1/4 cup marinara sauce (low-sugar, sodium-conscious brand)
- 1/4 cup shredded mozzarella cheese (reduced-fat)
- Salt and pepper to taste

Directions:

1. Preheat oven to 450°F (230°C). Line a baking sheet with parchment paper.
2. Prep the chicken: Pound the chicken breast to an even thickness of about 1/2 inch. Season with salt and pepper.
3. Prepare the breading: Combine breadcrumbs and Parmesan cheese in a shallow dish. In a separate dish, whisk the egg.
4. Bread the chicken: Dip the chicken in the egg, then coat evenly in the breadcrumb mixture. Press firmly to ensure good adhesion.
5. Bake the chicken: Place the breaded chicken on the prepared baking sheet. Bake for 20 minutes, or until cooked through and golden brown.
6. Add the sauce and cheese: Remove the chicken from the oven. Top each piece with 2 tablespoons of marinara sauce and 2 tablespoons of shredded mozzarella cheese.
7. Broil (optional): For extra browning and melted cheese, broil for 1-2 minutes, watching closely to avoid burning.
8. Serve: Enjoy your Baked Chicken Parmesan with a side of steamed vegetables or a small salad.

Nutritional Information: Calories: 400, Protein: 40g, Carbohydrates: 30g, Fat: 15g, Fiber: 3g, Sodium: 350mg

Tips:

- For even lighter breading, use a mixture of breadcrumbs and ground flaxseed or almond flour.
- Choose a low-sugar, low-sodium marinara sauce for better overall calorie and sodium control.
- Adjust the amount of marinara and cheese depending on your desired calorie intake.
- Consider using a lower-fat mozzarella cheese alternative like part-skim or string cheese.
- Serve with a whole-wheat pasta or brown rice for a complete meal.

Sesame Ginger Beef Stir-Fry

Cooking Time: 15 minutes | **Prep Time**: 10 minutes | **Total Time**: 25 minutes | **Serving Size**: 2

Ingredients:

- 1 pound flank steak, thinly sliced
- 1 tablespoon soy sauce
- 1 tablespoon rice vinegar
- 1 teaspoon sesame oil
- 1 teaspoon grated ginger
- 1 clove garlic, minced
- 1/2 teaspoon cornstarch
- 1 cup broccoli florets
- 1 red bell pepper, sliced
- 1 cup green beans, trimmed
- 1/2 cup chopped green onions
- 1 tablespoon toasted sesame seeds

Directions:

1. Marinate the beef: In a bowl, combine soy sauce, rice vinegar, sesame oil, ginger, and garlic. Add the beef and toss to coat. Marinate for at least 10 minutes, while prepping the vegetables.
2. Prepare the vegetables: Wash and chop the broccoli, bell pepper, and green beans. Trim the green onions. Set aside.
3. Cook the beef: Heat a large skillet or wok over high heat. Add a drizzle of oil (not included in calorie count) and swirl to coat. Once hot, add the beef and cook, stirring constantly, for 2-3 minutes until browned and cooked through. Remove from the pan and set aside.
4. Stir-fry the vegetables: Add another drizzle of oil to the pan. Add the broccoli and bell pepper and stir-fry for 2-3 minutes until crisp-tender. Add the green beans and stir-fry for another minute.
5. Thicken the sauce: In a small bowl, whisk together the cornstarch and 2 tablespoons of water to make a slurry. Return the cooked beef to the pan with the vegetables. Pour in the sauce and stir-fry for 1 minute until thickened.
6. Garnish and serve: Stir in the green onions and sesame seeds. Serve immediately with brown rice or quinoa for a complete meal.

Nutritional Information per Serving: Calories: 350, Fat: 10g, Carbs: 25g, Protein: 30g

Tips:
- Use a lean cut of beef like flank steak or skirt steak for lower fat content.
- Adjust the amount of soy sauce and rice vinegar to your taste preference.
- For a thicker sauce, add another tablespoon of cornstarch slurry, 1 tablespoon at a time, until desired consistency is reached.
- You can add other vegetables of your choice, such as carrots, snow peas, or zucchini.
- Serve with a side of low-sodium soy sauce for those who prefer more salty flavor.

Caprese Stuffed Portobello Mushrooms

Cooking Time: 20-25 minutes | **Prep Time**: 10 minutes | **Total Time**: 30-35 minutes | **Serving Size**: 1 portobello

Ingredients:

- 2 large portobello mushrooms, stems removed and gills scraped clean
- 1 tablespoon olive oil
- 1/2 teaspoon dried oregano
- 1/4 teaspoon garlic powder
- Salt and pepper to taste
- 1 cup cherry tomatoes, halved
- 1/2 cup fresh mozzarella cheese, thinly sliced
- 1/4 cup fresh basil leaves, chiffonade (thinly sliced)

Directions:

1. Preheat oven to 400°F (200°C). Line a baking sheet with parchment paper.

2. In a small bowl, combine olive oil, oregano, garlic powder, salt, and pepper. Brush the inside of each portobello mushroom with the mixture.

3. Place the mushrooms on the prepared baking sheet and bake for 10 minutes.

4. While the mushrooms bake, toss together the cherry tomatoes, mozzarella cheese, and basil in a bowl.

5. After 10 minutes, remove the mushrooms from the oven and evenly distribute the tomato mixture among the portobello caps.

6. Bake for an additional 10-15 minutes, or until the cheese is melted and bubbly.

7. Serve immediately, garnished with additional fresh basil if desired.

Nutritional Information per Serving: Calories: 200, Fat: 8g, Carbohydrates: 15g, Fiber: 4g, Sugar: 5g, Protein: 12g, Sodium: 250mg

Tips:

- For a vegan option, use dairy-free mozzarella cheese.
- To add more protein, top with a sprinkle of chopped nuts or cooked lentils.
- If you don't have fresh basil, you can use 1/2 teaspoon dried basil.
- Serve with a side of roasted vegetables or a salad for a complete meal.

Lentil and Vegetable Soup

Prep Time: 10 minutes | **Cooking Time**: 30 minutes | **Total Time**: 40 minutes | **Serving Size**: 4

Ingredients:

- 1 tablespoon olive oil
- 1 onion, chopped
- 2 carrots, chopped
- 2 celery stalks, chopped
- 2 cloves garlic, minced
- 1 teaspoon ground cumin
- 1/2 teaspoon ground turmeric
- 1/4 teaspoon ground black pepper
- 4 cups low-sodium vegetable broth
- 1 cup dry brown lentils, rinsed
- 4 cups chopped kale or spinach
- 1 (14.5oz) can diced tomatoes, undrained
- 1/4 cup chopped fresh cilantro (optional)

Directions:

1. Heat olive oil in a large pot over medium heat. Add onion, carrots, celery, and garlic, and cook until softened, about 5 minutes.

2. Stir in cumin, turmeric, and black pepper. Cook for another minute.

3. Add vegetable broth, lentils, and tomatoes (with their juices). Bring to a boil, then reduce heat and simmer for 20 minutes, or until lentils are tender.

4. Stir in kale or spinach and cook until wilted.

5. Season with additional salt and pepper to taste, if desired. Garnish with fresh cilantro (optional).

Nutritional Information per serving: Calories: 250, Fat: 3g, Carbs: 30g, Fiber: 8g, Protein: 15g, Iron: 4mg, Potassium: 400mg

Tips:

- For a thicker soup, mash some of the lentils against the side of the pot with a fork before adding the greens.
- You can substitute brown rice or quinoa for the lentils for a different texture.
- Feel free to add other vegetables, such as bell peppers, zucchini, or mushrooms.
- Store leftover soup in an airtight container in the refrigerator for up to 3 days.

SNACK RECIPES

Greek Yogurt Parfait

Cooking Time: 0 minutes | **Prep Time**: 5 minutes | **Total Time**: 5 minutes | **Serving Size**: 1 serving

Ingredients:

- 125g plain Greek yogurt (2% fat or non-fat)
- 50g mixed berries (fresh or frozen)
- 25g unsweetened granola
- 1/4 teaspoon ground cinnamon (optional)

Directions:

1. Gather your ingredients and prepare the workspace. Wash and dry all fruits. Measure out the yogurt, granola, and cinnamon (if using).

2. Assemble the parfait: In a glass or container, layer half of the Greek yogurt at the bottom.

3. Top with half of the mixed berries.

4. Sprinkle evenly with half of the granola.

5. Repeat steps 2-4 with the remaining yogurt, berries, and granola.

6. Dust with ground cinnamon for a warm flavor, if desired.

7. Enjoy immediately!

Nutritional Information per serving: Calories: 250, Fat: 5g, Saturated Fat: 2g, Carbohydrates: 25g, Fiber: 5g, Sugar: 10g, Protein: 20g

Tips:

- For a sweeter parfait, use a small amount of honey, maple syrup, or stevia to flavor the yogurt.
- Add a drizzle of nut butter for extra protein and healthy fats.
- Substitute the berries with other fruits like diced mango, pineapple, or kiwi.
- Use chia seeds instead of granola for added fiber and omega-3s.
- Make ahead of time: Assemble the parfait in jars or containers and store in the refrigerator overnight for a grab-and-go breakfast.

Vegetable Sticks with Hummus

Cook Time: None | **Prep Time**: 10 minutes | **Total Time**: 10 minutes | **Serving Size**: 1

Ingredients

- 1 medium carrot, washed and trimmed
- 1 medium cucumber, washed and trimmed
- 1 medium celery stalk, washed and trimmed
- 1 medium bell pepper, any color, washed and trimmed
- 1/4 cup plain hummus (check label for low-fat options)

Directions:

1. Prep the vegetables: Cut the carrot, cucumber, celery, and bell pepper into sticks or slices of similar size. Aim for thicker sticks for dipping convenience.

2. Assemble the snack: Arrange the vegetable sticks on a plate or divide them into individual containers for portion control. Place the hummus in a small bowl or container in the center.

3. Enjoy! Dip the vegetable sticks into the hummus and savor the healthy and satisfying flavors.

Nutritional Information per serving: Calories: 180, Fat: 3g, Saturated Fat: 0.5g, Carbohydrates: 24g, Fiber: 6g, Sugar: 6g, Protein: 4g, Sodium: 130mg

Tips:

- For variety, try different types of vegetables like broccoli florets, radishes, or sugar snap peas.
- Experiment with different flavored hummus options, but be mindful of added sugars and sodium content.
- Make sure the hummus is fresh and not past its expiration date.
- If you prefer a chilled snack, refrigerate the vegetables and hummus beforehand.
- Pair this snack with a glass of water to stay hydrated.
- Remember, portion control is key, so stick to the recommended serving size.

Apple Sandwiches

Prep Time: 5 minutes | **Cooking Time**: 0 minutes | **Total Time**: 5 minutes | **Servings**: 1

Ingredients:

- 1 medium apple, cored and thinly sliced
- 2 tablespoons unsweetened nut butter (almond, peanut, cashew, etc.)

Directions:

1. Wash and core the apple. Slice it thinly and evenly, discarding the core.

2. Spread 1 tablespoon of nut butter on one side of each apple slice.

3. Stack two apple slices together, nut butter sides facing each other, to create a "sandwich."

4. Repeat with the remaining apple slices and nut butter.

5. Enjoy immediately!

Nutritional Information per Serving: Calories: 180, Fat: 7g, Carbohydrates: 24g, Fiber: 4g, Protein: 3g, Sugar: 18g

Tips:

- For extra flavor, sprinkle the top of the "sandwich" with a pinch of cinnamon or chia seeds.
- If you prefer a sweeter snack, drizzle a small amount of honey or maple syrup on top.
- Use different types of nut butter for variety.
- Make sure to choose unsweetened nut butter for the lowest sugar content.
- Pair these sandwiches with sliced veggies or carrot sticks for added nutrients and crunch.
- Store leftover sandwiches in an airtight container in the refrigerator for up to 2 days. However, the apples may brown slightly.

Hard-Boiled Eggs with Avocado

Cooking Time: 12-15 minutes | **Prep Time**: 5 minutes | **Total Time**: 17-20 minutes | **Serving Size**: 1 person

Ingredients:

- 2 large eggs
- 1/2 ripe avocado, mashed
- 1/4 teaspoon lemon juice
- Salt and pepper to taste
- Optional: Pinch of red pepper flakes

Directions:

1. Cook the eggs: Bring a pot of water to a rolling boil. Gently lower the eggs into the boiling water and immediately remove the pot from heat. Cover and let the eggs sit for 12-15 minutes for perfectly hard-boiled eggs.

2. Cool and peel the eggs: While the eggs cook, prepare a bowl of ice water. Once cooked, transfer the eggs to the ice water bath and let them cool completely for 10-15 minutes. Peel the eggs carefully.

3. Assemble the dish: Slice the eggs in half or quarters. Divide the mashed avocado between two plates. Top each plate with the sliced eggs.

4. Season and enjoy: Drizzle with lemon juice and sprinkle with salt, pepper, and optional red pepper flakes. Enjoy!

Nutritional Information per serving: Calories: 246, Fat: 17g (of which 2g saturated), Carbs: 3g, Fiber: 3g, Protein: 12g, Cholesterol: 213mg, Sodium: 63mg

Tips:

- For easier peeling, add a teaspoon of baking soda to the boiling water with the eggs.
- Use ripe avocados for the best flavor and texture.
- Customize the flavors by adding a sprinkle of chopped herbs, a dash of hot sauce, or a drizzle of balsamic vinegar.
- Enjoy this dish with whole-wheat toast, baby spinach, or sliced tomatoes for a more complete meal.
- For an even lighter option, skip the lemon juice and use a smaller avocado (1/4).

Trail Mix

Prep Time: 5 minutes | **Cooking Time**: none | **Total Time**: 5 minutes | **Serving Size**: 1/4 cup

Ingredients:

- 1/4 cup raw almonds
- 1/4 cup raw walnuts
- 1/4 cup raw pumpkin seeds
- 1/4 cup unsweetened dried cranberries
- 1/4 cup unsweetened shredded coconut

Directions:

1. In a large bowl, combine all the ingredients.

2. Mix well to ensure even distribution.

3. Portion the trail mix into individual snack bags or airtight containers for easy on-the-go access.

Nutritional Information per Serving: Calories: 180, Fat: 10g (2g saturated), Carbs: 15g (5g fiber), Protein: 5g, Sugar: 7g (natural sugars from dried fruit)

Tips:

- For a sweeter mix, add a small handful of raisins or chopped dates. Be mindful of portion sizes as dried fruit can be high in sugar.
- For a crunchy texture, toast the nuts and seeds in a dry oven at 350°F for 5-10 minutes before adding them to the mix.
- If you like a touch of salt, sprinkle a small pinch of sea salt over the mix before portioning.
- Store the trail mix in an airtight container in a cool, dark place for up to 2 weeks.

Cottage Cheese with Pineapple

Cooking Time: None | **Prep Time**: 5 minutes | **Total Time**: 5 minutes | **Serving Size**: 1

Ingredients:

- 1/2 cup (125g) low-fat cottage cheese
- 1/4 cup (60g) fresh pineapple, diced
- 1/4 teaspoon ground cinnamon (optional)

Directions:

1. Gather your ingredients: Ensure you have all the ingredients measured and ready.

2. Combine cottage cheese and pineapple: In a small bowl, combine the cottage cheese and pineapple chunks. Mix gently until well combined.

3. Season with cinnamon (optional): If desired, sprinkle the ground cinnamon on top of the mixture for a warm and aromatic touch.

4. Serve and enjoy: Immediately consume your delicious and healthy snack.

Nutritional Information per serving: Calories: 140, Protein: 14g, Fat: 3g, Carbohydrates: 15g\, Fiber: 2g, Sugar: 12g

Tips:

- Use low-fat or fat-free cottage cheese for a lower calorie option.
- For a creamier texture, choose cottage cheese with a higher fat content.
- If you want the pineapple to be sweeter, let it sit for a few minutes before adding it to the cottage cheese.
- Substitute fresh pineapple with canned pineapple in 100% juice for convenience. Drain the juice before adding to the cottage cheese.
- Add a sprinkle of chopped nuts or seeds for extra crunch and protein.
- Enjoy your cottage cheese and pineapple as a post-workout snack, a light breakfast, or a satisfying afternoon treat.

Rice Cake with Cottage Cheese and Tomato

Prep Time: 5 minutes | **Cooking Time**: 0 minutes | **Total Time**: 5 minutes | **Serving Size**: 1

Ingredients:

- 1 round brown rice cake (30g)
- 1/2 cup (100g) low-fat cottage cheese
- 1 medium tomato, chopped (50g)
- Freshly ground black pepper, to taste

Optional Ingredients:
- Fresh herbs like basil or oregano
- A drizzle of balsamic vinegar or olive oil
- Spices like garlic powder or paprika

Directions:

1. Assemble: Spread the cottage cheese evenly over the rice cake.

2. Top it off: Arrange the chopped tomato over the cottage cheese.

3. Season: Sprinkle with freshly ground black pepper to taste.

4. Enjoy: Serve immediately.

Nutritional Information per Serving: Calories: 140, Total Fat: 2g, Carbs: 20g, Sugars: 4g, Protein: 10g, Sodium: 200mg, Fiber: 1g

Tips:

- For a warmer touch, toast the rice cake in a toaster oven for a minute before topping.
- Use low-sodium cottage cheese to further reduce sodium intake.
- Experiment with different types of tomatoes for variety, like cherry tomatoes or sun-dried tomatoes.
- If you prefer a creamier texture, mash the cottage cheese slightly before spreading.
- Feel free to add a dash of your favorite spices for additional flavor without impacting your weight loss goals.

Greek Yogurt Dip with Veggie Chips

Cooking Time: None | **Prep Time**: 5 minutes | **Total Time**: 5 minutes | **Serving Size**: 1

Ingredients:

- 1/2 cup plain Greek yogurt (2% fat)
- 1/4 cup chopped cucumber
- 1 tablespoon chopped fresh dill
- 1/4 teaspoon garlic powder
- 1/8 teaspoon onion powder
- Pinch of black pepper
- Pinch of salt (optional, taste first)
- Veggie chips of your choice (baked sweet potato chips, lentil chips, whole wheat pita bread slices, etc.)

Directions:

1. In a small bowl, whisk together the Greek yogurt, cucumber, dill, garlic powder, onion powder, black pepper, and salt (if using).

2. Taste the dip and adjust seasonings as desired.

3. Serve immediately with your preferred veggie chips.

Nutritional Information per Serving: Calories: 150, Fat: 5g, Carbohydrates: 10g, Fiber: 2g, Protein: 12g

Tips:

- For a thicker dip, drain some of the excess liquid from the cucumber before chopping.
- If you don't have fresh dill, you can use 1/4 teaspoon dried dill.
- Add a squeeze of lemon juice for a brighter flavor.
- Be mindful of portion sizes when enjoying chips, as they can be calorie-dense.
- If you're looking for even more protein, add a scoop of protein powder to the dip.
- Make a larger batch of the dip and store it in an airtight container in the refrigerator for up to 3 days.
- Experiment with different veggie chips to find your favorite flavor and texture combination.

Stuffed Mini Bell Peppers

Prep Time: 15 minutes | **Cooking Time**: 20 minutes | **Total Time**: 35 minutes | **Serving Size**: 8 mini bell peppers

Ingredients:

- 8 mini bell peppers, any color combination
- 1/2 cup cooked quinoa, rinsed and fluffed
- 1/4 cup chopped cucumber
- 1/4 cup chopped cherry tomatoes
- 1/4 cup crumbled low-fat feta cheese
- 1 tablespoon chopped fresh parsley
- 1 tablespoon lemon juice
- 1/4 teaspoon sea salt
- 1/8 teaspoon black pepper

Directions:

1. Preheat oven to 400°F (200°C). Line a baking sheet with parchment paper.
2. Prepare the bell peppers: Wash and dry the bell peppers. Cut them in half lengthwise, removing the seeds and membranes. Place them on the prepared baking sheet, open side up.
3. Make the filling: In a medium bowl, combine quinoa, cucumber, tomatoes, feta cheese, parsley, lemon juice, salt, and pepper. Mix well.
4. Stuff the peppers: Divide the filling evenly among the bell pepper halves. Gently press down to ensure the filling stays in place.
5. Bake: Bake for 20 minutes, or until the bell peppers are slightly tender and the filling is heated through.
6. Serve: Let the peppers cool slightly before serving. Enjoy as a snack, appetizer, or light meal.

Nutritional Information per serving: Calories: 75, Carbs: 7g, Fiber: 3g, Protein: 4g, Fat: 3g, Vitamin C: 100% RDI

Tips:

- For extra flavor, drizzle the filled peppers with a touch of olive oil before baking.
- If you prefer a firmer texture, leave the quinoa slightly undercooked before stuffing the peppers.
- To boost protein content, add cooked lean ground turkey or chicken to the filling.
- Experiment with different herbs and spices to personalize the flavor.
- To make this recipe vegan, substitute crumbled tofu for the feta cheese.

Edamame Salad

Cooking Time: 5 minutes | **Prep Time**: 10 minutes | **Total Time**: 15 minutes | **Serving Size**: 1 person

Ingredients:

- 1 cup frozen shelled edamame, thawed
- 2 cups mixed greens (romaine, spinach, kale, etc.)
- 1/2 cucumber, diced
- 1/2 bell pepper, diced
- 1/4 cup cherry tomatoes, halved
- 1 tablespoon red onion, diced (optional)
- 1 tablespoon olive oil
- 1 tablespoon lemon juice
- 1/2 teaspoon Dijon mustard
- Salt and pepper to taste

Directions:

1. Cook the edamame: Bring a pot of water to a boil. Add the edamame and cook for 3-5 minutes, or until tender. Drain and rinse with cold water.
2. Prepare the salad base: Wash and chop the mixed greens. Combine them in a large bowl.
3. Add the vegetables: Dice the cucumber, bell pepper, and cherry tomatoes. Add them to the bowl with the greens.
4. Make the dressing: In a small bowl, whisk together the olive oil, lemon juice, Dijon mustard, salt, and pepper.
5. Assemble the salad: Add the cooked edamame to the bowl with the vegetables. Pour the dressing over the salad and toss gently to combine.
6. Serve immediately. Enjoy your delicious and healthy Edamame Salad!

Nutritional Information per serving: Calories: 250, Fat: 8g, Carbs: 15g, Fiber: 8g, Protein: 17g, Iron: 10% DV, Vitamin C: 8% DV

Tips:

- For a spicier kick, add a pinch of red pepper flakes to the dressing.
- If you prefer a creamier dressing, add a tablespoon of plain Greek yogurt or mashed avocado.
- Feel free to add other low-calorie vegetables you enjoy, such as shredded carrots, radishes, or celery.
- Store leftover salad in an airtight container in the refrigerator for up to 2 days.

Greek Yogurt Bark

Prep Time: 10 minutes | **Cooking Time**: 0 minutes | **Total Time**: 10 minutes | **Servings**: 8-10 pieces

Ingredients:

- 1 1/2 cups plain, non-fat Greek yogurt
- 1/4 cup unsweetened applesauce
- 1/2 teaspoon vanilla extract
- 1/4 cup sliced fresh berries (strawberries, blueberries, raspberries)
- 1/4 cup chopped unsalted nuts (almonds, pecans, walnuts)

Directions:

1. Line a baking sheet with parchment paper.

2. In a medium bowl, whisk together the Greek yogurt, applesauce, and vanilla extract until smooth.

3. Spread the yogurt mixture evenly onto the prepared baking sheet in a thin layer, about 1/4-inch thick.

4. Sprinkle the berries and nuts over the top of the yogurt.

5. Place the baking sheet in the freezer for at least 3-4 hours, or until the bark is completely frozen solid.

6. When ready to serve, remove the bark from the freezer and break it into pieces.

Nutritional Information per Serving: Calories: 120, Fat: 2g, Saturated Fat: 1g, Carbohydrates: 14g, Fiber: 2g, Sugar: 8g, Protein: 12g

Tips:

- For an extra sweet treat, drizzle a small amount of melted sugar-free chocolate over the bark before freezing.
- You can use any type of fresh berries or nuts that you like.
- Make sure to use unsweetened applesauce to keep the overall sugar content low.
- If you don't have parchment paper, you can use a silicone baking mat instead.
- Store leftover bark in an airtight container in the freezer for up to 2 weeks.

Cucumber Slices with Tuna Salad

Cooking Time: None | **Prep Time**: 10 minutes | **Total Time**: 10 minutes | **Serving Size**: 1 person

Ingredients:

- 1/2 cucumber, thinly sliced
- 1 can (5oz) tuna in water, drained
- 1/4 cup plain Greek yogurt
- 1 tablespoon Dijon mustard
- 1/4 teaspoon dried dill
- Pinch of black pepper
- 1/4 red onion, finely diced (optional)
- 1 stalk celery, finely diced (optional)

Directions:

1. Wash and slice the cucumber: Wash the cucumber and slice it thinly using a mandoline slicer or knife. Arrange the slices on a plate.

2. Prepare the tuna salad: In a bowl, combine the drained tuna, Greek yogurt, Dijon mustard, dill, and black pepper. Mix well until evenly combined. If using, gently fold in the diced red onion and celery.

3. Assemble the bites: Top each cucumber slice with a heaping tablespoon of the tuna salad.

4. Serve: Enjoy immediately.

Nutritional Information per Serving: Calories: 220, Fat: 5g, Carbohydrates: 6g, Fiber: 2g, Protein: 25g, Sodium: 280mg (depending on tuna brand)

Tips:

- For extra flavor, squeeze a little lemon juice over the tuna salad.
- Add a sprinkle of fresh herbs like parsley or chives for garnish.
- If you prefer a creamier texture, use slightly more Greek yogurt or a blend of yogurt and light mayonnaise.
- For a touch of sweetness, add a teaspoon of chopped apple or grapes to the tuna salad.
- Store leftover tuna salad in an airtight container in the refrigerator for up to 2 days.

Roasted Chickpeas

Prep Time: 5 minutes | **Cooking Time**: 40-45 minutes | **Total Time**: 50 minutes | **Serving Size**: 1 cup

Ingredients:

- 1 cup dried chickpeas, rinsed and soaked overnight
- 1 tablespoon olive oil
- 1/2 teaspoon salt
- 1/4 teaspoon black pepper

Directions:

1. Preheat oven to 200°C (400°F).

2. Drain and rinse the soaked chickpeas. Pat them dry with a paper towel.

3. In a large bowl, toss the chickpeas with olive oil, salt, and pepper.

4. Spread the chickpeas evenly on a baking sheet lined with parchment paper.

5. Bake for 40-45 minutes, or until the chickpeas are golden brown and crispy, stirring occasionally.

6. Let the chickpeas cool slightly before serving.

Nutritional Information per serving: Calories: 160, Fat: 4g, Saturated Fat: 1g, Cholesterol: 0mg, Sodium: 30mg, Fiber: 8g, Protein: 14g, Carbohydrates: 20g, Sugar: 3g

Tips:

- For a different flavor, add your favorite spices to the chickpeas before baking, such as cumin, cayenne pepper, or paprika.
- You can also roast the chickpeas with a light coating of your favorite spray oil instead of olive oil.
- Store leftover roasted chickpeas in an airtight container in the refrigerator for up to 5 days.

Caprese Skewers

Prep Time: 10 minutes | **Cooking Time**: 0 minutes | **Total Time**: 10 minutes | **Servings**: 4

Ingredients:

- 16 cherry tomatoes, washed and halved
- 1 cup mini mozzarella balls
- 16 fresh basil leaves
- ¼ cup balsamic vinegar
- Freshly ground black pepper, to taste

Directions:

1. Thread a cherry tomato half, mozzarella ball, and basil leaf onto a skewer. Repeat with remaining ingredients, creating 16 skewers in total.

2. Drizzle balsamic vinegar evenly over the skewers. Season with black pepper to taste.

3. Serve immediately and enjoy!

Nutritional Information per serving: Calories: 120, Fat: 6g, Saturated Fat: 4g, Carbohydrates: 6g, Sugar: 4g, Protein: 8g, Sodium: 200mg

Tips:

- For a lighter option, use part-skim mozzarella cheese.
- Add variety by using different colored cherry tomatoes or adding a sprinkle of dried oregano.
- You can marinate the tomatoes in balsamic vinegar for 15 minutes before assembling the skewers for extra flavor.
- If you prefer a thicker balsamic glaze, simmer the vinegar in a small saucepan over low heat until it reduces by half.
- For a more filling option, pair your skewers with whole-wheat bread sticks or cucumber slices.

Almond Butter Energy Bites

Cooking Time: None | **Prep Time**: 10 minutes | **Total Time**: 10 minutes | **Serving Size**: 10-12 bites

Ingredients:

- 1/2 cup rolled oats
- 1/4 cup unsweetened shredded coconut
- 1/4 cup almond butter
- 1/4 cup pitted Medjool dates, chopped
- 2 tablespoons chia seeds
- 1 tablespoon honey
- 1/4 teaspoon cinnamon
- Pinch of sea salt

Directions:

1. In a large bowl, combine the rolled oats, shredded coconut, chia seeds, and cinnamon.
2. In a separate bowl, mash the dates with a fork until they become a sticky paste.
3. Add the almond butter, honey, and salt to the mashed dates and mix well until smooth.
4. Combine the wet and dry ingredients until well incorporated. The mixture should be sticky but hold its shape when pressed together.
5. If the mixture is too dry, add 1 tablespoon of water at a time until it reaches the desired consistency.
6. Use your hands to roll the mixture into 10-12 evenly sized balls.
7. Place the energy bites on a baking sheet lined with parchment paper.
8. Refrigerate for at least 30 minutes, or until firm.
9. Store leftover bites in an airtight container in the refrigerator for up to 5 days.

Nutritional Information per bite: Calories: 180, Fat: 8g, Carbs: 18g, Fiber: 3g, Protein: 5g

Tips:

- For a sweeter taste, you can add a few extra drops of honey.
- For a chocolatier flavor, mix in 1-2 tablespoons of unsweetened cocoa powder.
- If you don't have Medjool dates, you can use other dried fruits like raisins or apricots, but adjust the honey accordingly as they might be less sweet.
- Make sure to use natural almond butter without added sugar or unhealthy fats.
- Consider adding a sprinkle of hemp seeds or chopped nuts for extra protein and crunch.

Roasted Brussels sprouts

Prep Time: 10 minutes | **Cook Time**: 20-25 minutes | **Total Time**: 30-35 minutes | **Serving Size**: 2

Ingredients:

- 1 pound Brussels sprouts, trimmed and halved
- 1 tablespoon olive oil
- 1/2 teaspoon dried thyme
- 1/4 teaspoon kosher salt
- 1/4 teaspoon black pepper

Directions:

1. Preheat oven to 400°F (200°C). Line a baking sheet with parchment paper.

2. Trim the stem ends of the Brussels sprouts and halve them lengthwise.

3. In a large bowl, toss the Brussels sprouts with olive oil, thyme, salt, and pepper.

4. Spread the Brussels sprouts in a single layer on the prepared baking sheet.

5. Roast for 20-25 minutes, or until tender and lightly browned, flipping halfway through.

6. Serve immediately and enjoy!

Nutritional Information per serving: Calories: 50, Fat: 1g, Carbohydrates: 9g, Fiber: 4g, Sugar: 2g, Protein: 3g, Vitamin K: 75% RDI, Vitamin C: 80% RDI, Potassium: 10% RDI

Tips:

- For extra flavor, you can add a squeeze of lemon juice or balsamic vinegar after roasting.
- If you like your Brussels sprouts crispy, roast them for a few minutes longer.
- You can also use other herbs and spices, such as rosemary, paprika, or garlic powder.
- To make this recipe ahead of time, roast the Brussels sprouts as directed and then store them in an airtight container in the refrigerator for up to 3 days. Reheat them in the oven before serving.

Steamed Asparagus with Lemon

Prep Time: 5 minutes | **Cooking Time**: 5-7 minutes | **Total Time**: 10-12 minutes | **Servings**: 2

Ingredients:

- 1 bunch asparagus (about 12-15 spears)
- 1/2 lemon, zested and juiced
- Salt and pepper to taste

Directions:

1. Prep: Wash and trim the asparagus, removing about 1 inch from the woody ends.

2. Steam: Fill a pot with an inch of water. Bring to a boil over medium heat. Place a steamer basket in the pot, ensuring it doesn't touch the water. Add the asparagus to the basket. Cover and steam for 5-7 minutes, or until tender-crisp.

3. Season: Transfer the asparagus to a plate. Drizzle with fresh lemon juice, sprinkle with zest, and season with salt and pepper to taste.

4. Serve: Enjoy immediately as a side dish or light lunch.

Nutritional Information per Serving: Calories: 40, Fat: 0g, Carbs: 5g, Fiber: 2g, Sugar: 2g, Protein: 2g, Vitamin A: 40% DV, Vitamin C: 30% DV, Vitamin K: 50% DV

Tips:

- For thicker asparagus spears, increase the steaming time by 1-2 minutes.
- For a richer flavor, use a squeeze of olive oil instead of lemon juice.
- Add a pinch of crushed red pepper flakes for a bit of heat.
- This recipe is easily doubled or tripled to serve more people.

Quinoa Salad with Vegetables

Prep time: 10 minutes | **Cooking time**: 15 minutes | **Total time**: 25 minutes | **Servings**: 2

Ingredients:

- 1 cup quinoa, rinsed
- 1 1/2 cups water or vegetable broth
- 1/2 cucumber, chopped
- 1/2 red bell pepper, chopped
- 1/2 cup cherry tomatoes, halved
- 1/4 cup red onion, thinly sliced
- 1/4 cup fresh parsley, chopped
- 1 tablespoon olive oil
- 1 tablespoon lemon juice
- 1/2 teaspoon dried oregano
- Salt and black pepper to taste

Directions:

1. Rinse the quinoa in a fine-mesh sieve under cold water until the water runs clear.
2. In a saucepan, combine the quinoa and water or broth. Bring to a boil, then reduce heat, cover, and simmer for 15 minutes, or until the quinoa is cooked through and fluffy.
3. While the quinoa is cooking, prepare the vegetables. Chop the cucumber, bell pepper, cherry tomatoes, and red onion.
4. In a large bowl, combine the cooked quinoa, chopped vegetables, and parsley.
5. In a small bowl, whisk together the olive oil, lemon juice, oregano, salt, and pepper. Pour the dressing over the salad and toss to coat everything evenly.
6. Serve immediately or chill for up to 2 hours before serving.

Nutritional Information Per serving: Calories: 300, Fat: 4g, Carbs: 35g, Fiber: 6g, Protein: 8g

Tips:

- For a heartier salad, add cooked lean protein like grilled chicken or shrimp.
- You can also add other chopped vegetables of your choice, such as carrots, celery, or zucchini.
- To make the salad vegan, use vegetable broth instead of water and omit the parmesan cheese.
- For a spicier salad, add a pinch of red pepper flakes to the dressing.
- Store leftover salad in an airtight container in the refrigerator for up to 3 days.

Grilled Zucchini with Herbs

Prep Time: 10 minutes | **Cooking Time**: 10-12 minutes | **Total Time**: 22 minutes | **Serving Size**: 1 person

Ingredients:

- 1 medium zucchini (about 6 ounces)
- 1 tablespoon olive oil
- 1/2 teaspoon dried oregano
- 1/4 teaspoon dried basil
- 1/4 teaspoon garlic powder
- Pinch of salt
- Pinch of black pepper

Directions:

1. Preheat your grill or grill pan to medium-high heat.

2. Wash and trim the zucchini. Slice it lengthwise into 1/4-inch thick planks.

3. In a small bowl, whisk together the olive oil, oregano, basil, garlic powder, salt, and pepper.

4. Toss the zucchini slices in the herb mixture until evenly coated.

5. Place the zucchini slices on the preheated grill in a single layer.

6. Grill for 5-6 minutes per side, or until tender and slightly charred.

7. Serve immediately and enjoy!

Nutritional Information per serving: Calories: 50, Fat: 1g, Carbohydrates: 6g, Fiber: 1g, Protein: 1g, Vitamin C: 30% Daily Value, Potassium: 10% Daily Value

Tips:

- For extra flavor, marinate the zucchini in the herb mixture for 30 minutes before grilling.
- You can also use fresh herbs instead of dried.
- Serve the grilled zucchini with a squeeze of lemon juice or a dollop of plain Greek yogurt.
- To make this recipe vegan, use avocado oil instead of olive oil.

Cauliflower Rice Stir-Fry

Prep Time: 10 minutes | **Cooking Time**: 15 minutes | **Total Time**: 25 minutes | **Servings**: 2

Ingredients:

- 1 head cauliflower, riced (about 4 cups)
- 1 tablespoon olive oil
- 1 pound lean protein (chicken breast, shrimp, tofu), sliced or cubed
- 1 cup mixed vegetables (bell peppers, broccoli, carrots, snow peas)
- 2 cloves garlic, minced
- 1 tablespoon soy sauce
- 1 tablespoon rice vinegar
- 1 teaspoon sesame oil
- 1/2 teaspoon Sriracha sauce (optional, for spice)
- Salt and pepper to taste

Directions:

1. Prep: Wash and rice the cauliflower using a food processor, box grater, or knife. Wash and chop the vegetables and protein.
2. Cook the cauliflower: Heat olive oil in a large skillet or wok over medium heat. Add the cauliflower rice and cook for 5-7 minutes, stirring occasionally, until slightly softened.
3. Add protein: Push the cauliflower rice to one side of the pan and add the protein to the other side. Cook for 3-5 minutes, stirring occasionally, until browned.
4. Stir-fry vegetables: Add the vegetables and garlic to the pan with the protein and cook for 5-7 minutes, stirring frequently, until tender-crisp.
5. Combine and sauce: Combine the cauliflower rice, protein, and vegetables in the pan. In a small bowl, whisk together soy sauce, rice vinegar, sesame oil, and Sriracha (if using). Pour the sauce over the stir-fry and toss to coat everything evenly.
6. Season and serve: Season with salt and pepper to taste. Serve immediately, optionally garnished with fresh herbs like cilantro or green onions.

Nutritional Information per Serving: Calories: 330, Fat: 7g, Carbs: 25g (9g net carbs), Fiber: 5g, Protein: 20g

Tips:

- For additional protein, add a scrambled egg or cooked quinoa to the stir-fry.
- Adjust the vegetables to your liking. Other options include mushrooms, bok choy, or zucchini.
- To make it even lower in carbs, use coconut aminos instead of soy sauce.
- Store leftovers in an airtight container in the refrigerator for up to 3 days.

Spinach Salad with Strawberries and Almonds

Cooking Time: None | **Prep Time**: 10 minutes | **Total Time**: 10 minutes | **Serving Size**: 1

Ingredients:

- 4 cups baby spinach
- 1 cup sliced strawberries
- 1/4 cup sliced almonds
- For the dressing:
- 1 tablespoon olive oil
- 1 tablespoon balsamic vinegar
- 1 teaspoon Dijon mustard
- 1/2 teaspoon honey
- Salt and pepper to taste

Directions:

1. Wash and dry the spinach. Place it in a large bowl.

2. Add the sliced strawberries and almonds to the bowl.

3. In a small jar or bowl, whisk together the olive oil, balsamic vinegar, Dijon mustard, honey, salt, and pepper.

4. Pour the dressing over the salad and toss gently to coat all ingredients.

5. Serve immediately and enjoy!

Nutritional Information: Calories: 230, Fat: 7g, Carbohydrates: 18g, Fiber: 4g, Protein: 6g, Vitamin C: 80% DV, Iron: 15% DV

Tips:

- For a sweeter flavor, you can use a maple syrup or agave nectar instead of honey.
- Add a sprinkle of feta cheese or goat cheese for extra protein and tanginess.
- Use chopped walnuts or pecans instead of almonds for a different flavor profile.
- Serve this salad on its own or alongside grilled chicken, fish, or tofu for a complete meal.

Roasted Sweet Potatoes

Prep Time: 10 minutes | **Cooking Time**: 40-45 minutes | **Total Time**: 50-55 minutes | **Serving Size**: 1

Ingredients:

- 1 medium sweet potato
- 1 tablespoon olive oil
- 1/2 teaspoon paprika
- 1/4 teaspoon garlic powder
- 1/4 teaspoon black pepper
- Pinch of salt (optional)

Directions:

1. Preheat oven to 400°F (200°C).

2. Wash the sweet potato and pierce it a few times with a fork. You can leave the skin on for added fiber.

3. In a small bowl, mix olive oil, paprika, garlic powder, black pepper, and optional salt.

4. Rub the spice mixture evenly over the entire sweet potato.

5. Place the sweet potato on a baking sheet lined with parchment paper.

6. Roast for 40-45 minutes, or until tender when pierced with a fork.

7. Let cool slightly before slicing and serving.

Nutritional Information per Serving: Calories: 180, Carbs: 41g, Fiber: 6.6g, Protein: 4g, Fat: 0.3g, Vitamin A: 213% DV, Vitamin C: 44% DV, Manganese: 43% DV

Tips:

- For extra flavor, add a sprinkle of fresh herbs like rosemary or thyme before roasting.
- If you prefer a crispier texture, cut the sweet potato into wedges or cubes before roasting.
- If you're watching your sodium intake, skip the optional salt.
- Serve your roasted sweet potato with a light protein source like grilled chicken or fish, and a side of steamed vegetables for a complete and balanced meal.

Greek Cucumber Salad

Cooking Time: None | **Prep Time**: 10 minutes | **Total Time**: 10 minutes | **Serving Size**: 1

Ingredients:

- 1 English cucumber, peeled and thinly sliced (about 1 cup)
- 1/2 medium red onion, thinly sliced
- 1/4 cup cherry tomatoes, halved
- 1/4 cup crumbled feta cheese
- 1 tablespoon chopped fresh dill
- 1 tablespoon chopped fresh mint
- 2 tablespoons olive oil
- 1 tablespoon lemon juice
- 1/4 teaspoon dried oregano
- Salt and pepper to taste

Directions:

1. Combine: In a large bowl, combine the cucumber, red onion, and cherry tomatoes.

2. Dressing: In a small bowl, whisk together the olive oil, lemon juice, oregano, salt, and pepper.

3. Toss: Pour the dressing over the salad and toss to coat evenly.

4. Garnish: Sprinkle with feta cheese, dill, and mint. Serve immediately.

Nutritional Information per serving: Calories: 120, Fat: 6g, Carbs: 8g, Fiber: 2g, Protein: 3g

Tips:

- For a spicier salad, add a pinch of red pepper flakes to the dressing.
- If you don't have fresh herbs, you can use 1/2 teaspoon dried dill and 1/2 teaspoon dried mint.
- To make the salad ahead of time, prepare everything except the dressing and store it in the refrigerator for up to 2 hours. Add the dressing just before serving.

Stir-Fried Green Beans with Garlic

Prep Time: 5 minutes | **Cooking Time**: 5-7 minutes | **Total Time**: 12-14 minutes | **Servings**: 2

Ingredients:

- 1 pound fresh green beans, trimmed and snapped
- 2 cloves garlic, minced
- 1 tablespoon olive oil
- 1/4 teaspoon salt
- 1/4 teaspoon black pepper
- 1 tablespoon low-sodium soy sauce (optional)

Directions:

1. Prep the green beans: Wash and trim the green beans, removing the ends. Snap them into bite-sized pieces.

2. Heat the oil: In a large skillet or wok, heat the olive oil over medium-high heat until shimmering.

3. Sauté the garlic: Add the garlic and cook for 30 seconds, until fragrant but not browned.

4. Cook the green beans: Add the green beans and toss to coat with the oil. Cook for 3-5 minutes, stirring frequently, until the green beans are crisp-tender but still bright green.

5. Season and serve: Season with salt and pepper to taste. Add soy sauce, if desired, and toss to combine. Serve immediately.

Nutritional Information per serving: Calories: 70, Fat: 2g, Carbs: 8g, Fiber: 3g, Protein: 3g, Sodium: 100mg (depending on soy sauce amount)

Tips:

- For extra flavor, add a pinch of red pepper flakes with the garlic.
- To boost the protein content, add a cooked, lean protein like grilled chicken or tofu before serving.
- Serve over brown rice or quinoa for a complete meal.
- Store leftovers in an airtight container in the refrigerator for up to 3 days.

Broccoli Salad with Cranberries and Almonds

Prep Time: 10 minutes | **Cooking Time**: 0 minutes | **Total Time**: 10 minutes | **Servings**: 2

Ingredients:

- 4 cups broccoli florets, chopped
- 1/3 cup slivered almonds
- 1/3 cup dried cranberries
- 1/4 cup finely chopped red onion (optional, soak in cold water for 5 minutes to remove harshness)
- 2 tablespoons plain Greek yogurt
- 1 tablespoon light mayonnaise
- 1 tablespoon apple cider vinegar
- 1/2 teaspoon Dijon mustard
- Salt and freshly ground black pepper to taste

Directions:

1. Toast the almonds (optional): If you prefer toasted almonds, heat a dry skillet over medium heat. Add the almonds and cook, stirring frequently, until lightly golden and fragrant, about 3-5 minutes. Set aside to cool.
2. Prepare the broccoli: Wash and chop the broccoli florets into bite-sized pieces. You can steam them lightly for 2-3 minutes to soften them slightly, or leave them raw for a crunchier texture.
3. Combine the ingredients: In a large bowl, combine the chopped broccoli, toasted almonds (if using), dried cranberries, and red onion (if using).
4. Make the dressing: In a separate bowl, whisk together the Greek yogurt, mayonnaise, apple cider vinegar, Dijon mustard, salt, and pepper until smooth.
5. Assemble the salad: Pour the dressing over the salad ingredients and toss gently to coat everything evenly.
6. Chill and serve: Cover the salad and refrigerate for at least 30 minutes to allow the flavors to meld. Enjoy!

Nutritional Information per Serving: Calories: 250, Fat: 10g (of which 2g saturated), Carbohydrates: 15g (of which 5g sugar), Fiber: 5g, Protein: 8g

Tips:

- For a vegan option, use vegan mayonnaise or substitute the mayonnaise with mashed avocado.
- You can add a sprinkle of chopped fresh herbs like parsley or dill for extra flavor.
- If you prefer a sweeter salad, add a touch of honey or maple syrup to the dressing.
- Store leftover salad in an airtight container in the refrigerator for up to 3 days.

Mushroom and Spinach Sauté

Prep Time: 5 minutes | **Cooking Time**: 10 minutes | **Total Time**: 15 minutes | **Servings**: 1

Ingredients:

- 1 tablespoon olive oil
- 1 cup sliced button mushrooms
- 2 cloves garlic, minced
- 4 ounces fresh baby spinach
- 1/4 teaspoon salt
- 1/8 teaspoon black pepper

Directions:

1. Heat the oil: In a large skillet, heat the olive oil over medium heat.

2. Sauté the mushrooms: Add the mushrooms to the pan and cook, stirring occasionally, until softened and golden brown, about 5 minutes.

3. Add garlic: Stir in the garlic and cook for 30 seconds until fragrant.

4. Wilt the spinach: Add the spinach to the pan and cook, stirring constantly, until wilted and just tender, about 1-2 minutes.

5. Season and serve: Season with salt and pepper to taste. Serve immediately.

Nutritional Information: Calories: 78, Fat: 3.5g, Carbohydrates: 4.5g, Fiber: 2g, Protein: 5g

Tips:

- For added flavor, you can use different types of mushrooms, such as cremini, portobello, or shiitake.
- If you like a little heat, add a pinch of red pepper flakes.
- Serve this sauté over quinoa, brown rice, or whole-wheat pasta for a complete meal.
- You can also add a squeeze of lemon juice or a dollop of low-fat Greek yogurt for additional flavor and protein.
- Store leftovers in an airtight container in the refrigerator for up to 3 days.

Baked Eggplant Parmesan

Prep Time: 20 minutes | **Cooking Time**: 40 minutes | **Total Time**: 60 minutes | **Servings**: 4

Ingredients:

- 1 medium eggplant (about 1 pound), sliced into 1/2-inch rounds
- 1/4 cup whole wheat flour
- 1/4 cup panko breadcrumbs
- 1 teaspoon Italian seasoning
- 1/2 teaspoon garlic powder
- 1/4 teaspoon salt
- 1/4 teaspoon black pepper
- 2 large eggs, beaten
- 1 (14.5 oz) can crushed tomatoes, no sugar added
- 1/2 cup shredded low-fat mozzarella cheese
- 1/4 cup grated Parmesan cheese
- Fresh basil leaves, for garnish (optional)

Directions:

1. Prep the eggplant: Sprinkle both sides of the eggplant slices with salt and let them sit for 15 minutes. This helps draw out excess moisture, resulting in a less greasy dish. Rinse the slices and pat them dry with paper towels.
2. Prepare the coating: Combine the flour, breadcrumbs, Italian seasoning, garlic powder, salt, and pepper in a shallow dish.
3. Bread the eggplant: Dip each eggplant slice in the beaten egg, then coat evenly in the breadcrumb mixture.
4. Bake the eggplant: Preheat oven to 400°F (200°C). Line a baking sheet with parchment paper and arrange the breaded eggplant slices in a single layer. Bake for 20 minutes, flipping halfway through, until golden brown and tender.
5. Assemble the dish: Spread half of the crushed tomatoes in a 9x13 inch baking dish. Top with the baked eggplant slices, followed by half of the mozzarella cheese and half of the Parmesan cheese. Repeat with another layer of crushed tomatoes, eggplant, mozzarella, and Parmesan.
6. Bake and serve: Bake for 15-20 minutes, or until the cheese is melted and bubbly. Garnish with fresh basil leaves (optional) and serve immediately.

Nutritional Information per Serving: Calories: 350, Fat: 12g, Carbs: 30g, Protein: 25g, Fiber: 4g

Tips:

- For a crispier topping, broil the assembled dish for the last 2-3 minutes of baking.
- Use homemade or low-sodium store-bought crushed tomatoes for better control over sodium content.
- Substitute low-fat ricotta cheese for half of the mozzarella cheese for added protein and creaminess.
- Serve with a side salad or roasted vegetables for a complete and balanced meal.

Cucumber Avocado Salad

Prep Time: 10 minutes | **Cooking Time**: None | **Total Time**: 10 minutes | **Servings**: 1

Ingredients:

- 1 medium cucumber, peeled and sliced
- 1/2 ripe avocado, diced
- 1/4 red onion, thinly sliced
- 1/4 cup cherry tomatoes, halved
- 1 tablespoon fresh lemon juice
- 1 tablespoon olive oil
- Salt and black pepper to taste
- Optional garnish: Fresh cilantro leaves (not included in calorie count)

Directions:

1. Wash and slice the cucumber. You can slice it into rounds, half-moons, or even dice it depending on your preference.

2. Dice the avocado. Drizzle it with some lemon juice to prevent browning.

3. Thinly slice the red onion.

4. Halve the cherry tomatoes.

5. In a bowl, combine the cucumber, avocado, red onion, and cherry tomatoes.

6. Dress the salad with lemon juice, olive oil, salt, and pepper to taste. Toss gently to coat all ingredients.

7. Garnish with fresh cilantro leaves (optional).

Nutritional Information per serving: Calories: 240, Fat: 17g (of which 2g saturated), Carbohydrates: 8g (of which 4g fiber), Protein: 3g, Sodium: 120mg, Vitamin C: 14mg, Potassium: 350mg

Tips:

- For a creamier texture, mash a small portion of the avocado with the dressing before adding it to the salad.
- You can add a pinch of red pepper flakes for a bit of heat.
- If you don't have cherry tomatoes, you can use another type of tomato, such as diced roma tomatoes.
- To make this salad ahead of time, store the ingredients separately and assemble just before serving.

Roasted Cauliflower with Turmeric

Prep Time: 10 minutes | **Cooking Time**: 25-30 minutes | **Total Time**: 35-40 minutes | **Serving Size**: 2

Ingredients:

- 1 head cauliflower (about 1 pound), cut into florets
- 1 tablespoon olive oil
- 1 teaspoon ground turmeric
- 1/2 teaspoon smoked paprika
- 1/4 teaspoon black pepper
- 1/4 teaspoon garlic powder
- Pinch of salt

Directions:

1. Preheat your oven to 425°F (220°C). Line a baking sheet with parchment paper.

2. In a large bowl, combine the cauliflower florets with olive oil, turmeric, paprika, black pepper, garlic powder, and salt. Toss well to coat the cauliflower evenly.

3. Spread the cauliflower florets in a single layer on the prepared baking sheet.

4. Roast for 25-30 minutes, or until the cauliflower is tender and slightly browned, flipping halfway through cooking.

5. Serve immediately.

Nutritional Information per serving: Calories: 60, Fat: 0.5g, Carbohydrates: 8g, Fiber: 3g, Sugar: 2g, Protein: 2g, Vitamin C: 50% DV, Potassium: 10% DV

Tips:

- For extra flavor, drizzle the roasted cauliflower with a squeeze of fresh lemon juice or a sprinkle of chopped fresh herbs like parsley or cilantro.
- You can also add a pinch of cayenne pepper for a touch of heat.
- This recipe is easily doubled or tripled to serve more people.
- To make this recipe ahead of time, simply roast the cauliflower and store it in an airtight container in the refrigerator for up to 3 days. Reheat in the oven before serving.

Sautéed Swiss Chard with Garlic and Lemon

Prep Time: 5 minutes | **Cooking Time**: 10 minutes | **Total Time**: 15 minutes | **Servings**: 2

Ingredients:

- 1 tablespoon extra-virgin olive oil
- 1 bunch Swiss chard, stems removed and roughly chopped
- 2 cloves garlic, minced
- 1/2 teaspoon red pepper flakes (optional)
- Salt and black pepper to taste
- 2 tablespoons fresh lemon juice

Directions:

1. Prepare the chard: Wash the chard thoroughly and remove the stems. Roughly chop the leaves.

2. Sauté the garlic: Heat the olive oil in a large skillet over medium heat. Add the garlic and cook for 30 seconds, until fragrant.

3. Cook the chard: Add the chopped chard to the pan. Season with salt and pepper. Cook for 5-7 minutes, stirring occasionally, until the chard is wilted and tender.

4. Add flavor: Add the red pepper flakes (optional) and stir for another 30 seconds.

5. Finish with lemon: Add the lemon juice and stir to combine. Cook for an additional minute.

6. Serve: Remove from heat and serve immediately.

Nutritional Information per Serving: Calories: 45, Fat: 3.5g, Carbohydrates: 4g, Fiber: 1g, Sugar: 1g, Protein: 2g, Vitamin A: 25% DV, Vitamin C: 30% DV, Iron: 10% DV

Tips:

- For additional flavor, you can sprinkle the chard with Parmesan cheese or nutritional yeast before serving.
- If you prefer a milder flavor, reduce the amount of red pepper flakes or omit them entirely.
- This dish can be served as a side or part of a larger meal. It pairs well with lean protein, such as grilled chicken or fish, and whole grains, such as quinoa or brown rice.

SAUCES, DRESSINGS, AND DIPS

Greek Yogurt Tzatziki

Prep Time: 10 minutes | **Cooking Time**: 0 minutes | **Total Time**: 10 minutes | **Servings**: 2

Ingredients:

- 1/2 medium cucumber, peeled and grated (about 100g)
- 1 cup plain Greek yogurt, non-fat or 2% (200g)
- 1 tablespoon lemon juice (15ml)
- 1 tablespoon extra-virgin olive oil (15ml)
- 1 garlic clove, minced (1g)
- 1/4 teaspoon dried dill (0.5g)
- Pinch of salt and black pepper to taste

Directions:

1. Grate the cucumber: Use the large holes of a box grater and grate the peeled cucumber.

2. Drain the excess liquid: Place the grated cucumber in a clean dishcloth or cheesecloth and squeeze out as much liquid as possible. Transfer the squeezed cucumber to a bowl.

3. Combine ingredients: Add the Greek yogurt, lemon juice, olive oil, garlic, dill, salt, and pepper to the bowl with the cucumber.

4. Mix well: Stir until all ingredients are evenly combined.

5. Chill (optional): For a thicker consistency and more pronounced flavors, cover the bowl and refrigerate for at least 30 minutes.

6. Serve: Enjoy your tzatziki with fresh vegetables like carrots, cucumbers, bell peppers, or celery sticks. You can also use it as a spread on pita bread or as a sauce for grilled chicken or fish.

Nutritional Information per Serving: Calories: 140, Fat: 6g, Carbs: 6g, Protein: 12g, Fiber: 1g

Tips:

- Use a thicker Greek yogurt for a creamier dip.
- For a more intense garlic flavor, let the garlic sit in the yogurt for 10 minutes before adding the other ingredients.
- If you don't have fresh dill, you can use 1/2 teaspoon dried dill.
- You can use a food processor to grate the cucumber, but be careful not to over-process it as it can release more liquid.
- Store leftover tzatziki in an airtight container in the refrigerator for up to 3 days.

Guacamole

Prep Time: 5 minutes | **Cooking Time**: 0 minutes | **Total Time**: 5 minutes | **Servings**: 2

Ingredients:

- 1 ripe avocado, halved, pitted, and mashed
- 1/2 lime, juiced
- 1/4 red onion, finely diced
- 1 roma tomato, seeded and finely diced
- 1/4 cup fresh cilantro, chopped
- 1/2 jalapeno pepper, seeded and finely diced (optional, for spice)
- Salt and black pepper to taste

Directions:

1. Mash the avocado in a bowl until smooth.

2. Add the lime juice, red onion, tomato, cilantro, and jalapeno (if using).

3. Season with salt and pepper to taste.

4. Mix well until all ingredients are incorporated.

5. Serve immediately with whole-wheat pita bread, veggie sticks, or raw cucumber slices.

Nutritional Information: Calories: 180 per serving, Fat: 13g (7g monounsaturated), Fiber: 5g, Carbs: 7g, Sugar: 1g, Protein: 2g

Tips:

- Use a ripe avocado for the best flavor and texture.
- If you don't have fresh cilantro, you can substitute with parsley.
- For a creamier texture, add a tablespoon of plain Greek yogurt.
- To prevent browning, store unused guacamole in an airtight container with a layer of plastic wrap pressed directly onto the surface.

Homemade Salsa

Prep Time: 10 minutes | **Cooking Time**: 0 minutes | **Total Time**: 10 minutes | **Serving Size**: 1 cup

Ingredients:

- 2 medium roma tomatoes, seeded and diced
- 1/2 small red onion, finely diced
- 1 jalapeno pepper, seeded and finely diced (adjust for desired heat)
- 1/2 cup fresh cilantro, chopped
- 1 tablespoon fresh lime juice
- 1/4 teaspoon salt
- 1/8 teaspoon black pepper

Directions:

1. Combine all ingredients in a bowl and stir well to combine.

2. Taste and adjust seasonings as needed.

3. Cover and refrigerate for at least 30 minutes to allow the flavors to meld.

4. Serve chilled with your favorite low-calorie dippers like cucumber slices, bell pepper strips, or carrot sticks.

Nutritional Information per serving: Calories: 30, Fat: 0.5g, Carbs: 6g, Fiber: 2g, Sugar: 4g, Protein: 1g

Tips:

- For a smoother salsa, pulse the ingredients in a food processor a few times.
- You can also roast the tomatoes for a deeper flavor. Preheat the oven to 400°F (200°C). Toss the tomatoes with a little olive oil and salt, then spread them on a baking sheet and roast for 20-25 minutes, or until softened. Let cool slightly before using in the salsa.
- If you don't have fresh cilantro, you can substitute with parsley or another fresh herb.
- For a spicier salsa, leave some of the seeds in the jalapeno pepper.
- Store leftover salsa in an airtight container in the refrigerator for up to 3 days.

Hummus

Prep Time: 5 minutes | **Cooking Time**: 1 hour | **Total Time**: 1 hour 5 minutes | **Serving Size**: 1/4 cup (60g)

Ingredients:

- 1 cup dried chickpeas, soaked overnight
- 1/4 cup tahini
- 3 cloves garlic
- 1/2 lemon, juiced
- 1/4 cup water
- 1/2 teaspoon ground cumin
- 1/4 teaspoon sea salt
- 1/8 teaspoon black pepper

Directions:

1. Cook the chickpeas: Drain and rinse the soaked chickpeas. Add them to a large pot and cover with fresh water by 2 inches. Bring to a boil, then reduce heat and simmer for 1 hour or until tender. Drain and discard the cooking liquid.

2. Combine ingredients: In a food processor, combine the cooked chickpeas, tahini, garlic, lemon juice, water, cumin, salt, and pepper. Blend until smooth and creamy, scraping down the sides as needed. Add additional water, 1 tablespoon at a time, if needed to achieve desired consistency.

3. Serve: Enjoy your weight-loss hummus with sliced vegetables like carrots, cucumbers, bell peppers, or celery.

Nutritional Information per serving: Calories: 180, Fat: 6g, Saturated Fat: 1g, Polyunsaturated Fat: 2g, Monounsaturated Fat: 2g, Cholesterol: 0mg, Sodium: 300mg, Carbohydrates: 20g, Fiber: 5g, Sugar: 3g, Protein: 8g

Tips:

- For a smoother hummus, remove the skins from the chickpeas before blending.
- This recipe can be stored in an airtight container in the refrigerator for up to 5 days.
- Try adding a pinch of cayenne pepper for a spicy kick.
- Experiment with different herbs and spices for a variety of flavors.

Balsamic Vinaigrette

Prep Time: 5 minutes | **Cooking Time**: None | **Total Time**: 5 minutes | **Servings**: 2

Ingredients:

- 3 tablespoons extra virgin olive oil
- 2 tablespoons balsamic vinegar
- 1/2 teaspoon Dijon mustard
- 1/4 teaspoon dried oregano
- Salt and freshly ground black pepper to taste

Directions:

1. In a small bowl, whisk together the olive oil, balsamic vinegar, Dijon mustard, and oregano.

2. Season with salt and pepper to taste.

3. Serve immediately or store in an airtight container in the refrigerator for up to 5 days.

Nutritional Information per Serving: Calories: 70, Fat: 6g, Saturated Fat: 1g, Carbohydrates: 3g, Sugar: 2g, Sodium: 7mg

Tips:

- For a more flavorful vinaigrette, use a high-quality balsamic vinegar.
- Adjust the amount of vinegar and Dijon mustard to your taste preference.
- You can add a pinch of red pepper flakes for a bit of heat.
- This vinaigrette is also delicious drizzled over cooked chicken, fish, or tofu.

Lemon Herb Dressing

Prep Time: 5 minutes | **Cooking Time**: None | **Total Time**: 5 minutes | **Servings**: 2

Ingredients:

- 2 tablespoons extra virgin olive oil
- 2 tablespoons freshly squeezed lemon juice
- 1 teaspoon Dijon mustard
- 1/4 teaspoon dried oregano
- 1/4 teaspoon dried thyme
- 1/4 teaspoon dried parsley
- Pinch of black pepper
- Pinch of sea salt (optional, adjust to taste)

Directions:

1. In a small bowl or jar, whisk together all ingredients until well combined.

2. Taste and adjust seasoning as needed, adding more lemon juice, herbs, or spices to your preference.

3. Store in an airtight container in the refrigerator for up to 5 days.

Nutritional Information per Serving: Calories: 40, Fat: 3g, Carbohydrates: 2g, Sugar: 1g, Protein: 0g, Sodium: 30mg (depending on salt amount)

Tips:

- For a creamier dressing, add a tablespoon of plain Greek yogurt.
- If you don't have all the dried herbs, you can substitute with 1 tablespoon of fresh chopped herbs.
- This dressing can also be used on grilled chicken, fish, or vegetables.
- Be mindful of portion sizes, even with healthy dressings. Stick to the recommended serving size to manage your calorie intake.

Pesto Sauce

Prep Time: 5 minutes | **Cooking Time**: 0 minutes | **Total Time**: 5 minutes | **Servings**: 2

Ingredients:

- 2 cups packed fresh basil leaves, washed and dried
- 1/4 cup raw walnuts
- 1 garlic clove, peeled
- 1/4 cup low-fat feta cheese, crumbled
- 1/4 cup lemon juice
- 2 tablespoons extra virgin olive oil
- 1/4 teaspoon salt
- Freshly ground black pepper, to taste

Directions:

1. Toast the walnuts: (Optional) Preheat a small skillet over medium heat. Add the walnuts and toast for 2-3 minutes, stirring occasionally, until fragrant.
2. Combine ingredients: In a food processor, combine the basil, toasted walnuts (if using), garlic, feta cheese, lemon juice, olive oil, salt, and pepper.
3. Blend: Pulse the mixture until it reaches a desired consistency. You can stop to scrape down the sides if needed. Aim for a chunky or smooth texture, depending on your preference.
4. Taste and adjust: Taste the pesto and adjust seasonings as needed. Add more lemon juice, salt, or pepper to your liking.
5. Serve: Enjoy your pesto with whole-wheat pasta, roasted vegetables, grilled chicken or fish, or as a spread on whole-wheat bread.

Nutritional Information per serving: Calories: 180, Fat: 13g, Saturated Fat: 2g, Carbohydrates: 4g, Fiber: 1g, Protein: 6g, Sodium: 120mg

Tips:

- For a smoother pesto, add a tablespoon of water while blending.
- Store leftover pesto in an airtight container in the refrigerator for up to 3-4 days. You can also freeze it for longer storage.
- To make this recipe vegan, omit the feta cheese and use nutritional yeast instead.
- Explore different greens like spinach, kale, or arugula for variety.
- You can substitute walnuts with other nuts like pumpkin seeds, sunflower seeds, or almonds.

Asian Peanut Sauce

Prep Time: 5 minutes | **Cooking Time**: None | **Total Time**: 5 minutes | **Servings**: 2

Ingredients:

- 1/3 cup natural peanut butter (unsweetened and no added sugar)
- 2 tablespoons low-sodium soy sauce
- 2 tablespoons rice vinegar
- 1 tablespoon lime juice
- 1 clove garlic, minced
- 1/2 teaspoon grated ginger
- 1/4 cup water, or more to desired consistency
- Sriracha (optional, for added heat)

Directions:

1. In a small bowl, whisk together peanut butter, soy sauce, rice vinegar, lime juice, garlic, and ginger.

2. Gradually whisk in water until the sauce reaches your desired consistency. For a thinner sauce, add more water a tablespoon at a time.

3. Taste and adjust seasonings as desired.

4. Add a drizzle of sriracha for a spicy kick (optional).

Nutritional Information per serving: Calories: 140, Fat: 7g, Saturated Fat: 2g, Carbohydrates: 7g, Sugar: 4g, Protein: 4g, Fiber: 1g, Sodium: 280mg

Tips:

- Use natural, unsweetened peanut butter for the best flavor and to control sugar intake.
- Low-sodium soy sauce or tamari will help keep the sodium content in check.
- Taste the sauce before adding sriracha, as some peanut butters already have a bit of heat.
- For a thicker sauce, use less water or add a teaspoon of cornstarch mixed with a tablespoon of water and whisk it in until fully incorporated.
- This sauce can be stored in an airtight container in the refrigerator for up to 5 days.

Light Ranch Dressing

Ingredients:

- 1/4 cup (60ml) nonfat Greek yogurt
- 1 tablespoon low-fat buttermilk
- 1 tablespoon light mayonnaise
- 1/4 cup (60ml) chopped fresh dill
- 1 tablespoon chopped fresh chives
- 1/2 teaspoon dried onion powder
- 1/4 teaspoon garlic powder
- 1/8 teaspoon black pepper

Directions:

1. In a small bowl, whisk together the Greek yogurt, buttermilk, and mayonnaise until smooth.

2. Stir in the dill, chives, onion powder, garlic powder, and black pepper.

3. Taste and adjust seasonings to your preference.

4. Cover and refrigerate for at least 30 minutes to allow the flavors to meld.

5. Enjoy on your favorite salad!

Nutritional Information per serving: Calories: 35, Fat: 2g, Sodium: 130mg, Carbohydrates: 3g, Sugar: 1g, Protein: 1g

Tips:

- For a thinner dressing, add a tablespoon of water or low-sodium vegetable broth.
- If you don't have fresh herbs, you can substitute 1/2 teaspoon dried dill and 1/4 teaspoon dried chives.
- This dressing will keep in the refrigerator for up to 5 days.
- Remember, even light dressings can still add calories, so use them in moderation.

Cilantro Lime Dressing

Prep Time: 5 minutes | **Cooking Time**: None | **Total Time**: 5 minutes | **Serving Size**: 1/4 cup

Ingredients:

- 1/2 cup fresh cilantro leaves, chopped
- 1/4 cup fresh lime juice
- 2 tablespoons extra virgin olive oil
- 1 garlic clove, minced
- 1/4 teaspoon sea salt
- 1/4 teaspoon black pepper

Directions:

1. Combine all ingredients in a blender or food processor. Blend until smooth.

2. Taste and adjust seasonings as needed. You can add a pinch more salt, pepper, or a touch of honey for sweetness (adjust serving size information accordingly if adding honey).

3. Store in an airtight container in the refrigerator for up to 5 days.

Nutritional Information per Serving: Calories: 80, Fat: 6g (Monounsaturated), Carbohydrates: 3g (Sugar: 1g), Protein: 1g, Sodium: 30mg, Fiber: 1g, Vitamin C: 15% Daily Value

Tips:

- For a spicier dressing, add a small jalapeno pepper, seeded and chopped.
- If you don't have fresh cilantro, you can substitute 1 tablespoon dried cilantro, but the flavor will be less vibrant.
- This dressing is also delicious as a marinade for chicken or fish. Simply marinate for 30 minutes to 1 hour before cooking.

Batch Cooking Tips

Batch cooking is a fantastic strategy for those on a weight loss diet, as it allows you to prepare healthy meals in advance, saving time and ensuring that nutritious options are readily available when hunger strikes. Here are some batch cooking tips specifically tailored to a weight loss diet:

1. Plan Your Meals: Before you start batch cooking, take some time to plan your meals for the week. Consider incorporating a variety of lean proteins, whole grains, vegetables, and healthy fats to ensure balanced nutrition.

2. Choose Simple Recipes: Opt for recipes that are easy to prepare in large quantities and can be stored well. One-pot meals, soups, stews, and casseroles are excellent options for batch cooking.

3. Invest in Quality Storage Containers: Purchase a variety of high-quality storage containers in different sizes to accommodate your batch-cooked meals. Choose containers that are freezer-safe, microwave-safe, and stackable for easy storage.

4. Use Time-Saving Appliances: Utilize time-saving appliances such as slow cookers, pressure cookers (like Instant Pot), and sheet pans to streamline the batch cooking process. These appliances allow you to cook large quantities of food with minimal hands-on time.

5. Prep Ingredients in Bulk: Save time by prepping ingredients in bulk. Wash and chop vegetables, marinate meats, and portion out ingredients ahead of time, so they're ready to go when you start cooking.

6. Cook in Batches: Dedicate a specific day or time each week to batch cooking. Cook multiple meals at once, focusing on recipes that can be easily portioned and stored for later use.

7. Label and Date: Properly label and date each batch-cooked meal or ingredient to ensure freshness and avoid food waste. Include the name of the dish and the date it was prepared for easy identification.

8. Portion Control: When portioning out batch-cooked meals, use measuring cups, food scales, or pre-portioned containers to ensure accurate serving sizes. This helps prevent overeating and ensures that you stick to your weight loss goals.

9. Variety is Key: Keep things interesting by incorporating a variety of flavors, textures, and cuisines into your batch-cooked meals. Experiment with different spices, herbs, and sauces to add variety to your meals without adding excess calories.

10. Rotate Your Meals: To prevent boredom and maintain interest in your batch-cooked meals, rotate your menu regularly. Try incorporating new recipes and flavors each week to keep things fresh and exciting.

11. Stock Your Freezer: Take advantage of your freezer space by storing batch-cooked meals in portioned containers. This allows you to have a variety of healthy options on hand for busy days or when you're short on time.

12. Prep Snacks and Breakfasts: In addition to main meals, batch cook snacks and breakfasts to have nutritious options available throughout the week. Examples include overnight oats, energy balls, chopped vegetables with hummus, and hard-boiled eggs.

By implementing these batch cooking tips, you can streamline meal preparation, save time, and stay on track with your weight loss goals. With a little planning and organization, batch cooking can be a powerful tool for achieving and maintaining a healthy lifestyle.

Freezing and Storage Guidelines

Freezing and storage guidelines are crucial for maintaining the quality and safety of batch-cooked meals and ingredients. Here are some tips to ensure that your frozen foods remain fresh and delicious:

Freezing Guidelines:

➢ Cool Foods Properly: Allow cooked foods to cool to room temperature before freezing to prevent bacterial growth. Divide large batches into smaller portions for quicker cooling.

➢ Use Freezer-Safe Containers: Choose containers specifically designed for freezing, such as BPA-free plastic containers, glass containers with tight-fitting lids, or heavy-duty freezer bags. Make sure containers are labeled as "freezer-safe."

➢ Wrap Foods Well: Wrap foods tightly in plastic wrap, aluminum foil, or freezer paper to prevent freezer burn and maintain quality. For liquids or soups, use freezer-safe bags or containers with minimal headspace to prevent ice crystals from forming.

➢ Remove Excess Air: When using freezer bags, remove as much air as possible before sealing to prevent freezer burn and maintain freshness.

➢ Label and Date: Properly label each container or bag with the name of the dish and the date it was prepared. Use permanent markers or freezer-safe labels to ensure clarity.

➢ Follow Safe Thawing Practices: When ready to use, thaw frozen foods safely in the refrigerator overnight or use the defrost setting on your microwave. Avoid thawing foods at room temperature to prevent bacterial growth.

Storage Guidelines:

- Organize Your Freezer: Arrange frozen foods in your freezer in an organized manner, with labels facing forward and older items placed in front for easier access. Consider using stackable bins or shelves to maximize space.

- Maintain Proper Temperature: Keep your freezer at 0°F (-18°C) or below to ensure food safety and prevent spoilage. Use a freezer thermometer to monitor temperature regularly.

- Rotate Your Stock: Rotate your frozen stock regularly to ensure that older items are used first. Consider creating an inventory list to keep track of what's in your freezer and when it was prepared.

- Maximize Storage Life: Most cooked dishes can be safely stored in the freezer for up to 3-6 months, depending on the type of food and storage conditions. Follow recommended storage times for specific foods to maintain quality.

- Thaw Safely: Thaw frozen foods safely in the refrigerator, microwave, or cold water bath. Use thawed foods within 1-2 days and do not refreeze unless they have been cooked first.

- Discard if Needed: If frozen foods develop an off odor, flavor, or texture, or if there are signs of freezer burn (such as ice crystals or discoloration), discard them to avoid foodborne illness.

WEEK 1

Day 1:
Breakfast: Greek Yogurt Parfait
Lunch: Grilled Chicken Salad
Dinner: Grilled Lemon Herb Chicken

Day 2:
Breakfast: Vegetable Omelette
Lunch: Lentil Soup
Dinner: Baked Salmon with Dill Sauce

Day 3:
Breakfast: Quinoa Breakfast Bowl
Lunch: Turkey and Avocado Wrap
Dinner: Stir-Fried Tofu and Vegetables

Day 4:
Breakfast: Whole Grain Toast with Avocado and Egg
Lunch: Tuna Salad Lettuce Wraps
Dinner: Zucchini Noodles with Turkey Meatballs

Day 5:
Breakfast: Chia Seed Pudding
Lunch: Veggie and Hummus Wrap
Dinner: Vegetarian Chili

Day 6:
Breakfast: Smoothie Bowl
Lunch: Salmon and Asparagus
Dinner: Grilled Shrimp Skewers with Quinoa Salad

Day 7:
Breakfast: Egg Muffins
Lunch: Chickpea Salad
Dinner: Stuffed Bell Peppers

WEEK 2

Day 8:
Breakfast: Cottage Cheese Pancakes
Lunch: Greek Yogurt Chicken Salad
Dinner: Mushroom and Spinach Stuffed Chicken

Day 9:
Breakfast: Overnight Oats
Lunch: Vegetable and Tofu Stir-Fry
Dinner: Cauliflower Fried Rice

Day 10:
Breakfast: Egg and Veggie Breakfast Burrito
Lunch: Egg Salad Lettuce Cups
Dinner: Baked Cod with Tomato and Olive Relish

Day 11:
Breakfast: Zucchini Fritters
Lunch: Cauliflower Fried Rice
Dinner: Turkey and Vegetable Lettuce Wraps

Day 12:
Breakfast: Banana Walnut Overnight French toast Bake
Lunch: Turkey and Bean Chili
Dinner: Spaghetti Squash with Turkey Bolognese

Day 13:
Breakfast: Egg White Veggie Scramble
Lunch: Caprese Salad
Dinner: Cabbage and Beef Stir-Fry

Day 14:
Breakfast: Fruit and Nut Breakfast Bowl
Lunch: Veggie and Bean Burrito Bowl
Dinner: Lentil and Vegetable Soup

CONCLUSION

In wrapping up our exploration of a weight loss diet, it becomes evident that this journey is far more than a mere recalibration of caloric intake. It's a profound reimagining of our relationship with food, one that prioritizes health, vitality, and sustainable habits over fleeting fads or restrictive regimens. As we've navigated through a plethora of breakfast, lunch, and dinner options in our two-week meal plan, the underlying message is clear: achieving weight loss need not equate to bland, monotonous meals devoid of satisfaction or enjoyment.

Indeed, our culinary voyage has been a celebration of flavor, diversity, and creativity. From the vibrant hues of a Greek Yogurt Parfait to the aromatic allure of a Stir-Fried Tofu and Vegetables dish, each recipe beckons us to embrace the abundance of wholesome ingredients that nature offers. Through mindful meal planning, batch cooking, and strategic freezing and storage practices, we've uncovered the secrets to efficient, practical meal preparation without compromising on quality or taste.

Yet, beyond the realm of recipes and cooking techniques lies a deeper truth: sustainable weight loss is a holistic endeavor that transcends the confines of the kitchen. It encompasses lifestyle choices, mindset shifts, and a profound understanding of our bodies' needs. It's about cultivating a positive relationship with food—one rooted in nourishment, balance, and self-compassion.

In this journey, there are no shortcuts or quick fixes. Instead, it's a gradual evolution—a journey of self-discovery and empowerment. It's about learning to listen to our bodies, honoring their signals, and making choices that serve our long-term well-being. It's about finding joy in movement, savoring the simple pleasures of wholesome meals, and embracing the journey toward optimal health with open hearts and minds.

As we bid adieu to this exploration of a weight loss diet, let us carry forward the lessons learned—the importance of mindful eating, the value of nutritious foods, and the power of self-care. Let us approach our wellness journey with patience, resilience, and an unwavering commitment to self-improvement. And above all, let us remember that true transformation begins not with the number on the scale, but with the profound shift in perspective that comes from nurturing our bodies, minds, and spirits with love and intention.

FREQUENTLY ASKED QUESTION (FAQ)

What is a weight loss diet?
A weight loss diet is a structured eating plan designed to help individuals achieve their desired weight or body composition goals. It typically involves consuming fewer calories than the body expends, often through a combination of portion control, nutrient-dense foods, and increased physical activity.

What foods should I eat on a weight loss diet?
Focus on whole, minimally processed foods such as fruits, vegetables, lean proteins, whole grains, and healthy fats. These foods are rich in nutrients, fiber, and protein, which can help keep you feeling full and satisfied while supporting weight loss efforts.

Are there foods I should avoid on a weight loss diet?
Limit foods high in added sugars, refined carbohydrates, unhealthy fats, and excess calories. This includes sugary beverages, processed snacks, fried foods, and desserts. Instead, opt for nutrient-dense alternatives that nourish your body and support your weight loss goals.

How many calories should I eat to lose weight?
The number of calories needed for weight loss varies depending on factors such as age, gender, weight, height, activity level, and metabolic rate. Generally, creating a calorie deficit of 500 to 750 calories per day can lead to a safe and sustainable weight loss of about 1 to 1.5 pounds per week.

What are some effective strategies for weight loss?
In addition to following a balanced diet, incorporating regular physical activity, staying hydrated, getting adequate sleep, managing stress, and practicing mindful eating are all important components of a successful weight loss plan. It's also helpful to set realistic goals, track your progress, and seek support from friends, family, or a healthcare professional if needed.

Can I still enjoy my favorite foods on a weight loss diet?
Yes, it's possible to enjoy your favorite foods in moderation while on a weight loss diet. Incorporating occasional treats or indulgences can help prevent feelings of deprivation and promote a healthy relationship with food. The key is moderation and portion control.

How long will it take to see results on a weight loss diet?
The timeline for seeing results varies from person to person and depends on factors such as starting weight, adherence to the diet plan, and individual metabolism. While some people may notice changes in weight or body composition relatively quickly, others may experience a more gradual progression. It's important to focus on making sustainable lifestyle changes rather than seeking rapid results.

What should I do if I plateau or struggle to lose weight?
Plateaus are common during weight loss journeys and may occur for various reasons, such as metabolic adaptation, changes in activity level, or fluctuations in water retention. If you hit a plateau or struggle to lose weight, consider adjusting your diet, increasing physical activity, varying your workouts, managing stress, or seeking guidance from a healthcare professional or registered dietitian for personalized recommendations.

GLOSSARY

1. Calorie: A unit of energy used to measure the energy content of food and beverages. Calories are consumed through eating and drinking and expended through metabolic processes and physical activity.

2. Nutrient-Dense: Foods that provide a high amount of nutrients relative to their calorie content. Nutrient-dense foods include fruits, vegetables, lean proteins, whole grains, and healthy fats.

3. Portion Control: The practice of managing portion sizes to regulate calorie intake and promote healthy eating habits. Portion control involves being mindful of serving sizes and avoiding oversized portions.

4. Lean Protein: Protein sources that are low in saturated fat and calories. Lean protein options include chicken breast, turkey, fish, tofu, beans, lentils, and low-fat dairy products.

5. Whole Grains: Grains that retain all parts of the grain kernel, including the bran, germ, and endosperm. Whole grains are rich in fiber, vitamins, minerals, and antioxidants and include options such as brown rice, quinoa, oats, barley, and whole wheat bread and pasta.

6. Healthy Fats: Unsaturated fats that provide essential fatty acids and support heart health. Healthy fat sources include avocados, nuts, seeds, olive oil, fatty fish (such as salmon and mackerel), and nut butters.

7. Fiber: A type of carbohydrate found in plant-based foods that the body cannot digest. Fiber promotes digestive health, regulates blood sugar levels, and helps you feel full and satisfied. High-fiber foods include fruits, vegetables, whole grains, legumes, and nuts.

8. Metabolism: The process by which the body converts food and beverages into energy. Basal metabolic rate (BMR) refers to the number of calories the body burns at rest to maintain essential functions, while metabolism also includes the calories burned through physical activity and digestion.

9. Plateau: A period during a weight loss journey where weight loss stalls or slows despite continued efforts. Plateaus are common and may occur due to factors such as metabolic adaptation, changes in activity level, or fluctuations in water retention.

10. BMI (Body Mass Index): A measure of body fat based on height and weight that is used to categorize individuals into underweight, normal weight, overweight, or obese categories. While BMI can be a useful screening tool, it does not directly measure body fat percentage or account for factors such as muscle mass.

11. Hydration: The process of maintaining adequate fluid balance in the body. Staying hydrated is essential for overall health, proper bodily functions, and optimal metabolism. Recommended fluid intake varies based on factors such as age, gender, activity level, and climate.

12. Mindful Eating: The practice of being present and aware of the eating experience, including hunger and fullness cues, taste, texture, and satisfaction. Mindful eating encourages a non-judgmental approach to food and promotes a healthier relationship with eating.